Aging
with a
Vengeance

Aging
with a
Vengeance

Your Second
Fifty Years
Unleashed

Claudia Jean

Echo Ridge Publishing
La Costa, California

Echo Ridge Publishing
2270 Camino Vida Roble, #M
La Costa, CA 92009
760-931-9275
www.echoridge.com

Excerpts from "Becoming Diana Vreeland" in *Victoria Magazine*, November 2002. From *Diana Vreeland* by Eleanor Dwight. William Morrow, 2002. Copyright © 2002 by Eleanor Dwight. Reprinted by permission of HarperCollins Publishers Inc. William Morrow.
  Adapted list *Branding Yourself: How to Look, Sound & Behave Your Way to Success* by Mary Spillane, p. 163. Pan Books, 2000. Copyright © Mary Spillane *2000*. By permission of A. M. Heath & Co. Ltd.

Quantity sales: Special discounts are available on quantity purchases by corporations, associations, and others. For details, contact the "Special Sales Department" at the number above.

Illustrations by Dee Dawson, Newport Beach, California
Copyediting and proofreading by PeopleSpeak, Laguna Hills, California
Interior design and composition by Robert Goodman, Silvercat®, San Diego, California
Cover design by Michael Lynch, San Diego, California
Photography by James Jaeger, Vista, California

First Edition
        08 07 06 05 04 03   10 9 8 7 6 5 4 3 2 1

Library of Congress Cataloging-in-Publication Data

Jean, Claudia.
  Aging with a vengeance : your second fifty years unleashed / Claudia Jean. -- 1st ed. -- La Costa, Calif. : Echo Ridge Publishing, 2004.
      p. ; cm.
  Includes bibliographical references and index.
  ISBN: 0-9740958-2-6
  1. Aging--Social aspects. 2. Middle aged women--Psychology. 3. Middle aged women--Attitudes. 4. Aging--Psychological aspects. 5. Self-Actualization (Psychology) I. Title.
HQ1061.J432004   2003114204
305.26/2–dc22

Printed in the United States of America

Contents

Acknowledgments

*I*n every discipline there are rules—none more so than in writing. To those who read this book just for the content, enjoy. To those of you who know the rules, please understand that my editor, Sharon Goldinger of PeopleSpeak, is the best, most knowledgeable rule-enforcer in the world. Where this book has failed to meet strict professional standards, it has been my "after fifty the rules are only suggestions" mentality that ignored her pleas and cajoling. For instance, as a final compromise on the last pass through the book, we split the difference on the number of exclamation points. (I tend to want them everywhere!) That said, I could not recommend her more highly for her sense of humor and ability—and, in the end, her stamina—to put a polish on my words that was not there.

My daughter, Alison, deserves special recognition for her ability to work with me every day and not kill me. She also took care of all the computer wizardry that I refuse to learn. She's special in spite of me, not because of me!

Thanks also go to my assistant, Donna Worsley, for believing in this book and amplifying my efforts with hours of hands-on support.

Dee Dawson came into my life on a whim the week I was looking for a fashion illustrator. Why her experience as an illustrator came up we will never know, but I grabbed her, and her interpretations speak for themselves.

There is no more talented photographer than the incomparable James Jaegar. His professionalism and humor made it easy to look good.

Michael Lynch finessed his concept for the book cover from photo shoot to unfinished layout while having to listen to a myriad of people. The fact that he could please us all and never lose his cool speaks volumes!

Last, but certainly not least, is the handiwork of Bob Goodman. The final interior design of the book—its readability and its beauty—was lovingly orchestrated by a man who loves and lives his work. He is an award-winning human being as well as artist.

There is so much that I, the reader, took for granted while merely enjoying a good book that will never be the same since I have visited the travails of bringing this book to life. It doesn't take a village just to raise a child, it takes one to raise a book. My heartfelt thanks to one and all who made this experience so positive!

Preface

I'm Claudia Jean and I'm proud to say that I am seventy-two
years old. Yes, my photo is current! This news may give you a
surge of positive energy, maybe even hope, about your own
aging process. You may even wish to know my secret for being
so "well preserved."

It is really quite simple; I am actually only in my fifties.
What's my point? Stop lying about your age by taking years
off. If, instead, you add ten, fifteen, or even twenty years to
your age, people will be simply amazed and follow you anywhere to find out your secrets.

In truth, age is irrelevant. A sense of life is what you crave.
Being considered young for your age is what satisfies the
spirit. So, pick an age at random. You get to choose. Just be
aware, if you ask *my* age, I may want to astound and delight
you with the length of my life's journey!

Aging with a Vengeance reflects my personal plan for aging, a
plan that came about not because I have all the answers but
because I have had the great fortune to be mentored by fabulous women ahead of me on the journey to a well-lived life.
These women have inspired my own quest for a youthful old

age. They have mapped a path toward aging that makes each year *more* powerful, not less. To go gently, gracefully into the night would deny my very nature so I choose to age forcefully, with a vengeance. Most importantly, I *choose* to age. Let it happen or make it happen; either way, age happens. My chances for a strong, healthy second fifty years increase in proportion to my ability to plan for them.

Consider yourself among the fortunate to have survived long enough to reach this portion of your potential life cycle. You have luckily reached an age where you can no longer die young. You are probably aware that even a long life is far too short, and you certainly want to make the most of the time ahead.

In this book, shared insights await all those approaching their second fifty years as well as those nearing their third fifty years and everyone in between. Time flies with or without your input. Harness the energy. This book is about you. It is about me. It is about us, the sisterhood of second-fifty-year women.

As for me, I plan to live to be 120 (dramatic pause), then get shot by a jealous wife. A girl has to have a plan! When I present this philosophy to a group, I get one of two responses: (1) a collective groan at the pause, then laughter at the punch line, or (2) spontaneous clapping at the pause, then whoops at the punch line. By the time you finish this book, if you truly study the map laid out for you by the sisterhood, you will be in the group that not only claps for but also cheers a 120-year life span.

Agreed, aging brings issues, but one constant remains:

- I cared how I looked in my twenties!
- I cared how I looked in my fifties!
- And most certainly, I will care how I look in my eighties!

It is not our sense of style that is changing, it is our physical presence. We need to find like-minded women ready to raise their voices in unison. We are here! We continue to live by Helen Reddy's mantra, "I am woman, hear me roar," but the timbre has changed. Pick your decade: 40s, 50s, 60s, 70s, 80s, 90s. This message applies to all of us.

Like their younger counterparts, second-fifty-year women have one mission. *Be seen* at every age and do it with *attitude!* That is aging with a vengeance. If you are not seen, you cannot make a difference, and you are *meant* to make a difference. If it takes wearing a yellow feather boa, then so be it! Don't be ignored!

If you have already chosen to age gracefully, good for you. I, on the other hand, choose to join with those who age on purpose—with a vengeance. Because I believe in the power of numbers, I am inviting those of you still in the planning stages for the future decades of your life to give my plan a look. You are personally invited to join this army of women who have a great passion for life, a love of laughter, and a sense of self that leaves a positive impact.

Aging with a Vengeance addresses parallel issues—loving yourself unconditionally and proactive aging. Both start with self-esteem, a commodity that really gets tested if your journey through menopause includes shifting body parts and skin that stops snapping back. Self-esteem is your gift to yourself. It cannot be purchased from or given by someone else. Self-esteem is your value; it is what you contribute; it is how you will be perceived. In other words, you are responsible for defining yourself. Study successfully aging women on the path ahead of you to glean the personal secrets that have given them so much passion about this journey we call life.

The sisterhood of the over-fifty woman offers no excuses. It does offer insights that are meant to shine a light on the unknown, providing direction and understanding in our common human experience. The sisterhood also empowers us to step to the front of the line when we so desire.

While *Aging with a Vengeance* certainly speaks to those in transition through menopause—the most emotionally charged passage since puberty—this book's louder voice is actually to every postmenopausal woman, whatever her decade. Passing through menopause is not the end but the beginning of our ability to create an exceptional life. We are moving boldly forward toward the light of positive hope, warm promise, exceptional purpose, and yes, engaged roaring!

As in all change, you must "own" the process. You choose to grow or not. You choose to make a difference or not. There are no answers here for those who live as victims. If you are to learn from the sisterhood, you must commit to applying its secrets to your own life.

The power of this book lies in that it was written to you, one individual, to support your personal agenda. Are you most interested in your changing emotional dynamics or the physical issues of aging? Do you wish to turn inward or are you looking for knowledge to increase your external power? *Aging with a Vengeance* leads you on a quest for your inner power, gives tips on the external expression of that power in dress, and then shows you how to change the world around you. The secrets of the sisterhood let you chart your own journey. This is a time of differentiation, not homogenization.

Warning! These principles are not to be used as an excuse to make negative judgments about another human traveler. Use these principles to analyze and strategize your position but also note the positions of those around you. Do not confuse analysis with judging. Judging is childish name-calling and not allowed. Analysis is determining truth and truth is individual.

Understand your personal truth and you empower your life. Understand how your truth is but a thread in a larger human fabric of truth and you empower those around you. Take comfort from those with similar truths but learn from those whose truths are different.

Cheer for your second fifty years! Why? Because rules, as such, no longer exist. After fifty, the rules are only *suggestions*. We can confidently redefine what is appropriate because we have the advantage of experience to know what really matters. We know that taking care of ourselves first is not selfish but necessary. Being irreverent and unconventional becomes our gift to ourselves and to the world around us. Taking ourselves less seriously is serious business!

This book was written in part because of my frustration toward seemingly small but pervasive and persistent negative media reactions toward those in their second fifty years. Because they have a national platform for change and use it well, I am dedicating this book to the women of the media—Katie Couric, Oprah Winfrey, Diane Sawyer, Barbara Walters, and the rest.

My Dearest Media Leaders:

As a longtime fan, I wish to call an important issue to your attention. Your influence with your audience means that you inspire changes in society in ways no one else can. The topic? Aging.

Becoming old is a goal, not a sentence. Life is a one-way street, and we need to stop riding the brakes. To live another day means we become another day older. After many, many of these days, if we are lucky, we become not just old but very old. There is no other way.

The problem? Two quick examples will suffice. First, the media has a tendency to refer to "that certain age" or whisper an advanced age in hushed tones. Fifty-plus and shame are not conjoined twins. It's okay to be older. Being over fifty is powerful, not quiet, and it certainly should not be hidden in a cliché. Try saying "those in their second fifty years" for we still have much to accomplish.

A second example of the problem occurred recently when the beautiful and talented Rita Moreno appeared on the *Today* show. When she mentioned that she is seventy-one years old, Katie reacted, as many would, with shock that Rita would want anyone to know. Rita is rightfully proud of her age. Rita is what every seventy-one-year-old can hope to be. Living seventy-one full, wonderful years earns bragging rights, not shame. Hooray for Rita and all her foxy seventy-one-year-old "sisters"—and she has many.

This book is dedicated to all the women of the media because you are far too kind and involved with us, your audience, to have a conscious bias against aging. A few words from you as the occasions arise will tip the scales back in balance. It's not just about the baby boomers, it's about our mothers and grandmothers too. You see, there are fifty-three million women over the age of forty-five today, and the number is growing. We don't have a store or television program that claims us as its demographic, and we're a little riled up about it.

We are planning to take our power and our bank accounts where we are appreciated. All we ask is that you put in a kind word for us. Let us brag about our long lives. You do have the ability to change the world by making it safe to grow old. Oh, and by the way, Katie, we look forward to welcoming you into our ranks for your second fifty years. It's a great place to end up! Just ask Oprah, Diane, and Barbara. Oh, yes, and Rita!

Sincerely yours,
Claudia Jean

Now that we're all on the same page, I can promise you this: our value, our purpose, and our power as second-fifty-year women has never been more definable. Take what you already know to be true, add a measure of wisdom from those who journey ahead of you, and define the word *unleashed* for yourself. Prepare to create your personal definition of power for there is not one type but many. Come, join me as we discover the secrets of the sisterhood.

Part 1
<u>Be:</u> Your Inside Story

Remember the fairy tale ending, "And she lived happily ever after"? The truth is that much of the living in the "ever after" part does not qualify as happy. If you want your real ever after to be as close to a fantasy as humanly possible, you need to keep asking questions. You need to be curious about what has worked for someone else. Aging well means you need to load your wagon, so to speak, with support, experience, and tricks to empower you. When we meet, I will trade some of what I have in my wagon for some of what you have in your wagon. In other words, "Come play with me!"

The goal for your second fifty years, plain and simple, is this: Be seen. Part I addresses your inside reality, represented by the word *be*. Your outside presence, the part of you that is *seen*, follows in Part II. *Be* comes before *seen*. That is as it should be.

Turn the page and begin to find the stories or insights that speak to your heart. Add notes of your own. Individualize the book for yourself. *Be*.

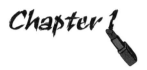

Chapter 1

Life Journey: Being Born Is Terminal

*I*f you are born, you will die. Does that seem too harsh? Get over it. Step into the truth, not around it. Embrace life's continuum; your birth assures your death. Acknowledging your eventual demise is your beginning, not your end. Acceptance of this fact assures that you are ready, first, to honor the age you are and then, second, to anticipate and strategize for the ages you will become.

Being born does not guarantee that you will grow old. Growing old is a treasure of great value. Become grateful for the gift. You or someone you know has lost a child to death's hold. You may have had friends who died in their teens and others as young adults, never reaching the ripe "old age" of fifty. Would you not choose to watch those loved ones grow old and gray with you rather than die so young?

Eventually, if you are lucky, you will face the issue of your personal aging process and your own mortality. A day comes when you finally are aware that, no matter how much you dig your heels in, you will one day be old. But *plan* to be old? Why?

The answer is control. You wanted control as a child; you want it even more now. You wanted control as a teenager and as a young adult; you want it even more now. The concept of aging may make you feel out of control, but here is the good news: for the rest of your life, you *can* take control. Drop the denial and embrace your strengths at each stage, and growing old successfully can become your greatest accomplishment.

Attitude Matters

Gaining control starts with your attitude. A recent study published in the *Journal of Personality and Social Psychology* has shown that *looking forward* to growing old adds 7.5 years to the length of your life.[1] Suzanne Kunkel, Ph.D., director of the Scripps Gerontology Center at Miami University and coauthor of the study, found that having a positive attitude toward aging was a more significant determinant of added years than quitting smoking, exercising, or controlling your cholesterol and blood pressure.

Planning to become old is a fabulous investment in your future, but in addition, when you plan for your tomorrows, today becomes incredible in and of itself. Aging with a vengeance means that you hug the promise of today while you expect many, many tomorrows.

Are changes to be expected as you age? Absolutely. Your physical strength at fifty-five is less than it was at forty-five but more than it will be at sixty-five. Accept it! Your sixty-five-year-old self will be stronger than you will be at seventy-five. The relativity is what is important, not your absolute strength. Appreciate your strength for today rather than mourn the loss from yesteryear for there is recompense: everything you give up in physical strength comes back to you in the currency of experience. *Plan* to have great experiences at every age. Vow to live in the strength of today, however strong.

A great line from the 1994 movie *The Shawshank Redemption* says it all: "Get busy living, or get busy dying."[2] Which will *you* choose—living or dying? Your choice determines your attitude. When you choose to live, you *choose* to age. Now, do it with a vengeance! *Plan* to create a legacy of focused vitality through all your years to come. Live on purpose, today, tomorrow, and every day after.

Life Stages

A woman's life can be divided into three stages with an important transition between each stage. These life stages bring differing issues and rewards. An understanding of these stages will help you maximize your own strengths and improve your interactions with your family and friends. (The ages are approximate.)

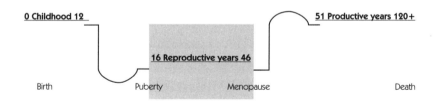

Life stages

Birth and death, the first and the last events of life, have a lot in common. Neither is in your control and both are typically a little messy and unscripted. Nature follows its own course, but your entry into the world assures your eventual exit. Your story and the difference you make, however long or short your life, is everything in between. It is therefore prudent to *wish* for more years, *plan* for more years, *expect* more years.

As the reader of this book, you are probably somewhere near the end of the reproductive years or beyond. A short visit to your earlier stages can clarify your future.

Stage One—Childhood

Childhood is a time of innocence. Modern psychology can define expected behaviors at each level of development, but children are generally emotionally free and accepting. As a child, you were blissfully unaware of sexuality, gender, or race. You were friends with all who wanted to play, and having fun seemed to be your main responsibility. You went from point A to point B at top speed, not always in a straight line. You laughed and squealed for no particular reason except that you could. What exuberance! Around twelve years of age that all changed.

Transition One—Puberty

Puberty is a time of predictable unpredictability. What a molting. What confusion and emotional upheaval it caused for both your parents and yourself. How sullen you often were. Your parents wondered what happened to their wonderful child. In fact, their child had disappeared. According to research reported in *Newsweek*, both in February and May 2000, as a teen you didn't just "molt" but experienced major changes in both hormones and brain physiology.[3] It has been found that during puberty a secondary laying down of gray matter over the brain causes all manner of strange behavior. The first time you experienced this laying down of new gray matter was at age two, with the result that your perceptions and behavior changed radically, producing the notorious "terrible twos." At puberty, perceptions and behavior changed just as radically for the same reasons, but by then you were larger and even more difficult to direct.

What were your parents to do except try to understand, hang on, and not overreact? At this stage, a parent's greatest directive is to try to keep their adolescents from killing themselves with drugs or alcohol or by driving too fast. Sadly, not all teenagers survive this transition.

Stage Two—The Reproductive Years

Between twelve and sixteen years of age, you entered a reproductive stage that is your lot for about the next thirty years. What responsibility and pressure this stage brings. These years are filled with mating, birthing, and attempting to raise good citizens, all while living with a boiling cauldron of hormones that have the ability to override both your best interests and logical decisions. The intensity of managing your chemistry is often confusing. The term "raging hormones" was not coined lightly.

The reproductive years involve using your power to create new life, build new businesses, expand political forces, and engineer a new world. These years are exciting, enervating, and yes, exhausting. Logically, might you not look forward to a second fifty years that could be less charged, more relaxed?

Transition Two—Menopause

Relief from the pressures of the reproductive years looms on your horizon, but this relief requires one more huge passage—menopause, or as I call it, "de-pubescence." At menopause, all the hormonal changes you went through in puberty are now revisited in reverse. Hormones still rage, but what was turned on in puberty must now turn off and does so in fits of random production over the course of several years.

While hormones made you *reproductive,* understand that the loss of these hormones will leave you potentially more *productive.* Sadly, the period between your reproductive years and your productive years is often confusing, conflicted, and a twisted journey unique to each individual. There is no set physiological switch or timetable.

✦ *"Menopause" versus "The Change"*

Previous generations euphemistically referred to menopause as "the change" but the baby boomer generation unabashedly uses the word "menopause." Issues once whispered about are now put on magazine covers and television specials for the world to see. Today, menopausal women feel so much more aware and informed.

Does knowledge about the journey through menopause make it easier? Articles are written; the subject and the word itself are not taboo. We are more intellectually enlightened, but the physical passage through menopause is often still a complete shock.

Similar stories abound, but since I found no volunteers for this segment, I make the following point using my own transition.

- In my 20s, I weighed 125 pounds.
- In my 30s, I weighed 135 pounds.
- In my 40s, I weighed 145 pounds.

Do you see a pattern here? At five feet eight inches I was comfortable with these incremental changes. A few additional pounds rounded out my shape and minimized soft crinkles as I got older. I reasonably expected that in my fifties I would weigh 155 pounds. No such luck! In the course of one year, as menses ceased and without increasing my caloric intake, I reached 170 pounds. Some say the body has a mind of its own after thirty, but in my experience, the body actually *loses* its mind completely after fifty!

None of my eating habits had changed; I was not taking in more calories. What was happening? Simple genetics. A lucky few do not gain weight at this stage, but if your genetics are so programmed, you will suffer the indignity of becoming that fuller figured middle-aged woman you were so sure you would never become. Sorry, it is what it is. Punish yourself or hug yourself—it is your choice. As for me? I choose to hug my "fluffier" but still fabulous self.

At my height, 125 is too thin, 145 comfortable. The truth is that these weights were "setpoints." Today, as in my younger years, I can either act reasonably and easily maintain my weight or I can deny myself most oral delights, cut my calories to 800 per day, and artificially reduce. If I stop dieting, I immediately go back to my age-appropriate, genetically determined, new setpoint. The beauty of setpoints is that we seldom gain beyond them. Relax into your new body for it is preparing to assist you to a healthy second fifty years.

But twenty-five pounds? Menopause, shmenopause, I just went through "the change." So much for being so smug. Mom's generation had it right.

✦ Weighing In

It is common to gain two dress sizes during menopause. Size twos become sixes. Size tens become fourteens. Even those who are not destined to gain weight report a new distribution to their curves. These changes have a purpose. Fat cells migrate to your hips for a reason. According to Debra Waterhouse, in her book *Outsmarting the Midlife Fat Cell* just when your hormonal cycle is shutting down, your new fat distribution surrounds your organs and gives off a low level of estrogen in an effort to ease your journey to the other side of reproduction.[4] Don't despair; those pounds that come on so suddenly at menopause tend to disappear just as stealthily in your early eighties, again without changing your normal routine or eating habits. It's something to look forward to—you will actually regain the figure of your youth if you will just be patient.

The weight I gained going through menopause is the same weight I carry today, five years later. My new setpoint is 170 pounds. There is a formula attempting to measure obesity called the body mass index (BMI). To find your BMI, first, divide your weight in pounds by your height in inches. Next, divide that result by your height again. Finally, multiply that number by 703.

BMI = Weight in pounds ÷ height in inches ÷ height in inches x 703

For example, here's how I figured my BMI.

My current BMI = (170 ÷ 68 ÷ 68) x 703 = 25.85
My premenopause BMI = (145 ÷ 68 ÷ 68) x 703 = 22.04

Find your own BMI: ____ ÷ ____ ÷ ____ x 703 = _____

A score between 20 and 25 means you are a healthy weight. A BMI of 25 to 30 is considered overweight. Do you see that according to the scale, a BMI of 25 is considered both healthy and unhealthy? Look at your whole health picture, such as blood pressure and family history, not just your weight. My BMI is over 25, my health otherwise perfect. Now what?

If a twenty- to thirty-pound weight gain is nearly universal through menopause, does it not follow that there is a natural purpose to that gain? Indeed, Dr. Annette Colby, R.D., reports that "if you are over 65 years of age, a BMI of 29 does not appear to be unhealthy and may even be a useful energy reserve in the case of illness."[5] Eureka! The body knows how to increase your chances for a healthy long life. It is possible that gaining a little bit toward that number each year is also healthy, if that is your genetic calling. Logically, the same weight cannot be considered unhealthy at sixty-four and magically healthy at sixty-five. If your BMI was healthy going into menopause and you are at a stable weight after menopause, just love your new self. Eat healthy, exercise a bit, and let your body be your guide. It intrinsically knows how to give your specific genetic code its best chance for survival.

✦ *Offer Support*

Before we move on to the third stage, we need to look at one more important point. We second-fifty-year women need to be especially aware and supportive of our friends, neighbors, and family members who have both transitions—puberty and menopause—occurring under one roof. Offer them respite from the seeming insanity. Offer promises of peace on the other side. It is just conjecture, but science may find out, in time, that there is actually a third laying down of gray matter at menopause just as at age two and at puberty. People in major transitions, whether as a two-year-old child, a pubescent teen, or a menopausal adult, benefit from the gentle wisdom of those who understand from experience that "this too shall pass."

Stage Three—The Productive Years

The move from your reproductive to your productive stage is eventually accomplished. Now you enter wonderful years, unfettered by the ups and downs of hormones. Bless the end of menses. Remember the first trip you took when you didn't have to count the days and take feminine products along with you? This absolute freedom is just one more reason to embrace this stage of life.

Now you discover the fabulous secret of the third stage of life: in the place of the innocence and joy of childhood, third stagers have experience and wisdom—and joy. Without all those reproductive pressures, life is suddenly peaceful. You have a long timeline ahead of you to just enjoy what is really important, surrounding yourself with people you adore. Now, mountains are much more easily turned into molehills—and you can even flatten most of the molehills. You don't "sweat the small stuff" because you know what is important. That is peace.

In the third stage, you face your life with a steady eye on maybe fifty more years of this kind of peace. As a productive woman, you relax, let go of the past, maximize the gift of living today, and, given scientific advances, rejoice in your potential to productively make a difference until the ripe old age of 120.

In what way are these years productive? In all the ways that matter! At this age, when you properly honor yourself and your point in history, you have the opportunity to shape the generations behind you while shining respect on those ahead of you. What is your reward? You open yourself to being taught how to age well, age long, and age with unabashed passion! Plus, you get a second chance.

✦ *Setting Things Right*

The productive years are the age of setting things right. Remember all the mistakes you made while raising your children? Parents make amends to their children by being loving grandparents to their grandchildren, especially when those grandchildren are teenagers. In fact, be a surrogate grandparent to all the teenagers in your sphere.

Parents often have a hard time letting go of their maturing children. As these young adults emerge, older adults best fulfill their destiny by providing the teenagers unconditional love and regard. Honor teenagers' individuality and their personal sense of self as they emotionally disconnect from their parents. This acceptance is your richest gift to future generations. Encourage their best selves to emerge by unswerving belief that these teenagers are the greatest creatures on the face of the earth.

My grandmother Tessie would privately tell all her grandchildren, whatever their abilities, that they were her favorite. We knew that she told all of us the same thing, but we felt great about it anyway. (Of course, in my heart of hearts, I am quite sure that I *really* was her favorite.) A huge part of my belief in myself is founded in the fact that Grandma believed in me even more. She shaped the futures of her brood of grandchildren with her unconditional love and acceptance.

Set limits on children's behavior but adore the individual openly. You cannot spoil a child by loving with an unconditional heart. In the end, you impact future generations because your grandchildren learn to grandparent from you. That is immortality enough.

✦ *Judge Not*

Harsh judgments toward the young give aging a bad name. Rather than criticize the expression of each generation's personal definition, be charmed by it. Every generation has to do something to make the older generations react. This rebellion is psychologically necessary. Boomers had the Beatles, long hair, hip-hugging bell-bottoms, and worse. Dreadlocks, piercings, and tattoos all represent physical expressions by current "emerging adults."

While a rebelling child's parent may overreact, you, the grandparent, can relax about the whole issue because you know something to be true: what this group is doing to shock their parents will eventually be topped by what their children (your great-grandchildren) will do to terrify them. You know the next generation will come up with something.

Rather than criticize, be a voice of reason. Call on your own youthful "rebellion." Recognize and acknowledge the youth on their interpretation of their generational statement. Share your personal generational statement and those of their parents. Were you a flapper? Did you dare bob your hair? Did you date men in zoot suits? Did you dance in five-day marathons? Did you live in short-shorts? Did you follow the Grateful Dead? Share your stories of bending the rules. Bending is necessary for maturing.

At this point, you can discuss the difference between costuming style and lifestyle. A strange haircut, shocking clothes, or even a tattoo won't kill you, but smoking, underage drinking, and drugs can. Clarify the difference. With a sense of humor, spend time discussing what styles they may be able to expect from the generation they will produce.

While at an airport, I noticed a boy, approximately twelve years old, waiting alone for a flight. He sported a four-inch, spiked Mohawk haircut. He wore a dog collar with a chain that hung down to and hooked through his belt loop. Baggy shorts, threatening to fall off his hips, and a torn muscle shirt completed the outfit. I was fascinated by his ability to so perfectly define himself at this young age and saw him as an excellent representative of his generational separation. As I mused to myself about his "costume," what did I see? A fifty-plus "hippie" with long hair and scruffy clothes approached this young boy and proceeded to berate his choice of attire. It was a case of the pot calling the kettle black. Most of the boomer hippies outgrew their rebellious style and reconnected to middle-class American mores and attitudes. Children *should* set new standards. Adults should grow up. I wish I had spoken up. My grandmother would have.

If you really want to strike terror in the heart of youth, there is a gentle way to accomplish your mission: compliment them. One fine summer day, outside a sandwich shop, I encountered a group of five young teenagers done up in amazing generational costume. My favorite had a pile of six- to eight-inch coiled dreadlocks on the top of his head while the sides and back were buzz clipped. His natural hair color was black but his dreadlocks were bleached blond and looked rather like a pile of snakes. His clothes were equally provocative. He was hard to ignore so I didn't try. I approached the group and told them I was honestly impressed with their creativity. I told them that in my generational breakout time in the 1960s, my friends and I had pushed the envelope and couldn't, at the time, believe there was anything left for a new generation to use to uniquely define itself.

My final comment? "You are all so creative and look fabulous. I'm really impressed! I just wonder what on earth is left for your kids to do to make their own statement." I could see the light of recognition in their eyes. They understood that what goes around, comes around. There is, in the end, balance in the universe.

✦ Finding the "Gold" in the Golden Years

The productive years are not just about what you can do for others. The second fifty years holds a wonderful treasure for those ready to receive it.

Your productive stage is indeed more powerful than your reproductive stage because you understand the importance of hugging the young, valuing yourself, and honoring your elders. This emotional balance, addressed in coming chapters, creates the "gold" of the golden years. It will become the most precious commodity in your bag of tricks.

Are there issues with growing old? Absolutely. Your body will decline by degrees. If you have visited your internist recently, you may have filled out a questionnaire that lists what seems like hundreds of potential issues involving the frailty of the human biological system. The list starts with "Please check all that apply," then proceeds something like this:

Ulcer	Stroke	High blood pressure	Arthritis
Hyperthyroid	Hypothyroid	High cholesterol	Rash
Cancer	Diabetes	Coronary disease	Osteoporosis
Glaucoma	Anemia	Asthma	Leg cramps
Spastic colon	Hepatitis	Liver disease	Back pain
Kidney disease	Dizziness	Macular degeneration	Bleeding problems

Unnerving, isn't it?

Relax. Seldom does one individual experience the doctor's list of ailments in its entirety. Rather, this list is a menu of possibilities that your genetic package will or will not succumb to. Most of us go through life with an issue here and an issue there but not an issue everywhere! If you make healthful living decisions regarding smoking, drinking, eating, sleeping, and exercising, many ailments are only textbook scenarios. Many perfectly healthy individuals in their eighties, nineties, and beyond are still going strong. You have every reason to expect to reach a very old age as vital, healthy, and truly alive.

Aging is not a disease. Believe it, enjoy it, live it. Still, eventually the end comes.

Death

Death is a fact. Eventually, you will come to the end of your journey. You depend on a combination of health, genetics, and fate to postpone your own final call as far into the future as possible. After all, you have so much to accomplish.

Do I personally have a guarantee of a full second fifty years? Of course not, but accepting my own inevitable end is all in the *spin*. Genetically, my family lives until they die. That is, we have little cancer, no heart attacks, no Alzheimer's disease, no arthritis, no osteoporosis. When we do die, it is typically by stroke. I have chosen to embrace the medical terminology for the probable cause of my demise—"cerebral event." See the difference in attitude? When I go, it will be an *event!* The dictionary defines *event* as an important happening or occurrence. That's good enough for me. I comfortably accept my end as part of the package we call life and will "party on" until that final *event*, whatever it may be.

✤ *Strategy for Your Event*

What about *your* final event? Whether it's a notice in the news-paper, a somber funeral, or a rowdy gathering of all your friends, what will people remember about you? What would you like said about you at your final event? This speech, if you plan it now, can become your agenda for a well-lived life because fabulous things cannot be said about you if you never quite get around to being fabulous.

Defining fabulous is as easy as reading the obituaries. You will learn from people you have never met how to live a well-spent life. If something strikes you as a beautiful compliment that you wish could be said about you, write it down. Change genders if necessary. For instance, consider this excerpt from an obituary in the *San Diego Union Tribune:* "When . . . left us, at age . . . , the world that [s]he enlivened was made immeasurably poorer. We miss [her] searching eyes that reflected [her] own bemused delight. Even if you did not know who [s]he was, you would be aware that [s]he was a person of significance. Over the years [s]he gained authority, learned how to eliminate, retaining only the essence."[6]

Fill in your name and select some ripe old age. Now, how would you live the rest of your life so this paragraph would be accurate?

Here's another example that shows that one does not need to be politically powerful to exude power. Read what one family wrote on the anniversary of their mother's death:

Dearest Mom,

One year after your passing, we honor and celebrate your life! We lovingly remember your many wonderful qualities, especially your keen sense of humor and quick wit, your radiant smile, your vibrant personality and zest for life, your warmth and sensitivity, and your compassionate loving soul. You shared your beautiful spirit with family, friends, and even strangers—all who knew you, loved you! Daily we were showered with the countless blessings of your unconditional love. Though we can no longer see you, you are with us still. You will always be more than a memory—you are a living presence in our daily lives. You live inside our laughter and our tears, our dreams and aspirations. Nothing can separate us, not time, not space, not even death. You will always be an integral part of our lives! With much love now and forever . . .[7]

Was she *just* a mom? You decide.

This concept will be revisited and expanded in chapter 4. For now, start your own collection of phrases that you wish to define your legacy. This exercise is not about dying but rather about living your life on purpose. Many great things can and will be said about you, especially when you plan!

✦ Grieve Well

But death brings grief. Should you deny grief? No, embrace it because grief is its own reward.

Currently, American behavior toward the dying process is undergoing an encouraging shift. Rather than institutionalizing the event, families are coming together to embrace the final days of their loved one's lives through hospice and home care. Bodies of the deceased are no longer covered and hurried from the room. Time is being spent with death, and grief is being felt rather than avoided.

You see, grief is the end of every true love story. Someone always has to go first. It is the human condition. Whether one lives to be 5 or 105, life is too short.

Grief is a reward, not a punishment. You grieve because you have loved. Those who do not love do not grieve for where there is no bond, there is no pain. Live your life so you will someday be grieved for. Meanwhile, embrace your ability to grieve deeply and grieve well because you also love deeply and love well.

The lesson here is simple but profound: if you are born, you will die. Prepare to honor all your ages and all your stages as you experience the chapters to come. Great age is indeed a valuable gift.

Chapter 2

Ageism: Getting beyond "Old"

*I*n my late twenties, a girlfriend's mother admonished us for spending far too much time in the sun. She cautioned us that as we got older we would come to regret our burn-and-peel routine, as it would prematurely age our skin. We both responded that it wouldn't matter how we looked when we got older. Having a great tan now was all that was important.

She looked me right in the eye and said, "Do you seriously think I don't care how I look today?" That was the first time I actually tried to picture myself as "older," and her challenge did rebalance my thinking somewhat. I agreed that I would probably care how I looked when I was an "old" woman like her. Looking back, I realize this beautiful woman was only in her early forties. Today, I see forty as just a beginning. Who keeps moving this perception of what is old?

In fact, every female over the age of ten is an "old" lady to someone. Those chronologically behind us see us as old. On the other hand, those ahead of us see us as young and perhaps naïve. We egocentrically insist that the age we are is the only age that counts. Since there's a high probability I'll succeed in reaching my personal goal, to live a very long life, I need to acknowledge that what I call "old" describes nothing but a position on the continuum of life. Seeing others as old diminishes the value of everyone ahead of me on that line. If I refuse to honor those ahead of me, those who have already been where I am, then I have no right to expect honor from those behind me.

It is not so grievous that the young disparage the old but that those old enough to know better do so. In my business, I go to the major clothing markets several times a year. It's exciting and exhausting. With thousands of vendors, multiple thousands of products, huge crowds, and permission to spend unbelievable amounts on clothes, it's an experience of wonderful guilt-free shopping!

One fall, during a break on the second day of such a trip, I was seated next to a lovely "older than me" woman who owned a shop in the Midwest. She had a great passion for her boutique, and we laughed about mutual issues in our businesses. When I mentioned my love for my oldest customers, those in their eighties and nineties, she abruptly started demeaning "older" women. I was stunned at her vitriol because she seemed to be in her early seventies herself. She had no perception of her own position on the aging continuum. This woman, whose boutique was geared toward an older demographic, identified with me, twenty years her junior, but not with those only ten to fifteen years older than she.

Being versus Feeling

You have certainly thought it, and you have probably said it: "I know I am getting older, but I don't *feel* any older." What is this nearly universal disconnect between the physical reality and the mental perception of aging? Welcome to the greatest, most profound secret of the sisterhood: the "inner girl."

The Inner Girl

Who is this inner girl? She is the part of you who consistently gives you a sense of youth and immortality. I have been aware of my own inner girl since my midthirties. In her eyes, I have unlimited potential and am eternally young. I really prefer to listen to her view of my future. What role does she play in my psychology and how can I use her to maximize my potential in my second fifty years?

Let me share one example of the way she speaks to me. My favorite Olympic sport is women's gymnastics. The sport is very, very physically demanding and I love watching it so much that I plan my schedule around the televised events. As the competition unfolds in front of me I emotionally experience every vault, dismount, and jump these athletic young women perform. A peculiar phenomenon occurs. I actually *feel* that if I just got off the couch, worked out a bit, and gave it a try, I could vault, dismount, and jump too! Never fear, the part of me that does the *thinking* is oh-so-well aware that that's impossible. Still, the potential to physically excel presented by my inner girl excites me.

You may already recognize your own inner girl. She represents your emotional age. Often that age is not a general figure but an actual year. When I tell you that my inner girl happens to be eighteen (on a very mature day), it explains a lot about how I view the world. When I honor my inner girl, my emotional age, I also take steps to protect the body she has at her disposal so I can try a few of the wonderful things she suggests.

If you are not already in touch with your own inner girl, try to define how old you experience yourself in your dream state. Typically, when dreaming, we "view" both our parents and ourselves as young adults, no matter what our respective chronological ages are.

If you still cannot identify your emotional age, try this exercise. Picture yourself on a beautiful tropical island. The sound of seabirds and waves mixes with the wonderful smell of salt air. Your porch swing creaks gently as you almost imperceptibly rock. The sun is setting into one of the most brilliant palettes of orange and red you have ever experienced. The balmy seventy-degree evening folds you in its arms. You have just experienced the most amazingly happy day you have ever lived. How old are you—not you the dreamer, but you within the dream? You're a young adult, right?

Popular psychologist John Bradshaw was responsible for many of us learning to identify our "inner child" and helping advance our understanding of early trauma and subsequent healing.[1] Even if you have never met your inner child, you can still meet and greet your inner girl. She is probably not just in her teens, twenties, thirties, or forties, but she has a specific age. How old is she? Define her for yourself. Mine is young, but I have been introduced to other inner girls ranging from age ten to thirty-five and even fifty. Women with older inner girls describe themselves as having been mature, "old souls" even as children, but they still have a definable younger self in their later years.

This inner girl speaks from our subconscious. She is that part of us that fights back against dire diagnoses of illness and survives in the face of horrible disasters. She does not accept "the final answer" until she agrees that it is time for life to end.

There is no right or wrong age for your true self. Your emotional age, this younger sense of self, is the powerhouse that successful second-fifty-year women have harnessed for themselves. Your emotional age expressed as your inner girl is a true Fountain of Youth. Respond to her, embrace her. She is your best friend.

Grandma

In my midthirties, I had a conversation with my wonderful Grandma Tessie, who was then in her late eighties. "Grandma," I said, "my kids are thirteen and ten years old now. I distinctly remember how I felt when I was their ages. Mom and Dad were adults and I felt safe because they had answers. I look at my kids and it scares me to death because I have no answers. I feel like I am only eighteen years old myself. *When do I get to feel like an adult?*"

Grandma's reply rings in my ears to this day, "Oh honey, I'm only twenty-one! Adulthood is mostly an illusion. I am constantly shocked by my reflection in the mirror and wonder who on earth hit that woman with the ugly stick."

I protested that I thought she was one of the most beautiful women I had ever known. Couldn't she see how loved she was by all the young people who were always at her house? (In fact, our whole family would agree that Grandma was *the* definition of "unconditional love." Everyone who met her became family and called her "Grandma.")

"Oh, I accept all that," she replied, "but sitting here looking out around me, I am not a wrinkled old woman. I am only twenty-one. It is only when I see something I want on top of the TV and I go to get it that I find my mind is already across the room, but my rear end is still on the couch! You will probably never be over eighteen. It's small comfort, but your parents didn't have any more answers than you do now."

Grandma knew her inner girl and she defined mine for me. Do you hear the promise? Your inner girl does not age with your body. She stays eternally young. Like Grandma, you may be confused by your reflection in the mirror as you get older, but how you *feel* toward yourself and your potential *will not change* until your subconscious agrees that your body has run its course. Again, aging is a biological process, not a mental process—not just for you but *for every woman ahead of you.*

Since my inner girl is eighteen years old, and I will take this feeling to my grave, how do I define myself? How do I balance this young driving force with the actual age I give the census bureau? Both my emotional age and my biological age have value and meaning. Neither should be denied or diminished.

Age versus Experience

While attending my first writer's conference I met two women who showed me the importance of both definitions of age. My very first contact was with a beautiful young writer who has had the great fortune to have already published seven novels. What an achievement! Our conversation drifted to *Aging with a Vengeance.* When people hear that I feel positive about getting older, they readily divulge their ages. This beautiful woman revealed that she had just been traumatized by her thirty-fifth birthday. I spent a few moments encouraging her to embrace her age and emphasized to her that the nearly twenty years since my own thirty-fifth birthday were undoubtedly my most productive and powerful. I assured her that she had such a head start for her age she would achieve rewards that, looking back, would make the whole journey seem fabulous. I also assured her that, unbelievably, we older women have little desire to go back in time. I doubt she believed me completely, but someday in the future if she remembers my words, she will know exactly what I meant.

The very last woman I met at this same conference was Phyllis, a renowned author, lecturer, and writing instructor. At a writer's conference, questions about one's work are polite even between a successful author and a first-time hopeful. I described my wish to change the face of our aging process by honoring that inner girl I knew and loved. Phyllis immediately responded, "You're absolutely right. I'm only in my twenties. No, actually, I am twenty-two."

The difference in our chronological ages immediately disappeared and we became eighteen- and twenty-two-year-old "sisters." Phyllis, very youthful and svelte, mentioned that she was seventy-four years old. I asked her, "You have exactly twenty years on me. Would you go back to fifty-four?" Her response was immediate and strident, "Absolutely not!"

Does this mean that if we second-fifty-year women woke up one morning with our former twenty-year-old bodies that we would disclaim them? Maybe. We are not willing to return to the limited experience of that twenty-year-old self nor do we wish to revisit the hormonal turmoil we have already left behind. Where we are is *better* than where we were.

So how do we account for this wealth of years? It obviously has high value if we are not ready to trade it in for our former youth. The ultimate gift of the sisterhood is that we can say, first to each other and then to those under fifty who fear the aging process:

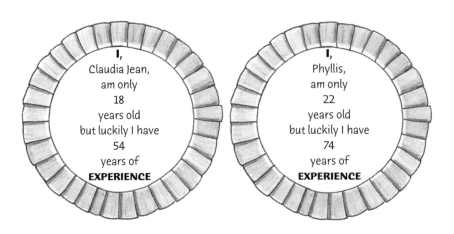

Now it is your turn!

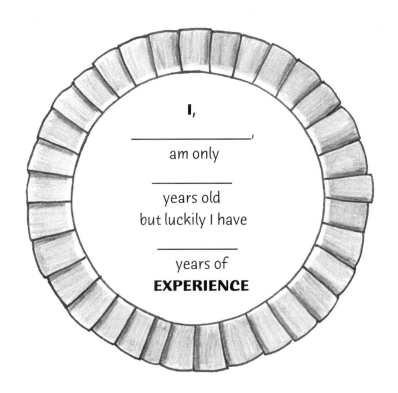

The True Fountain of Youth

Do you see that our eighteen- and twenty-two-year-old inner selves never change? These inner girls represent our emotional ages and are eternal. Our sense of humor, our wish to have fun, our belief that great opportunities still await, even our sense of irreverence permeates our being throughout our lives. Our fifty-four- and seventy-four-year-old *physical* selves will continue to advance—if we are lucky. It takes another year to be a year wiser and to have another year of experience.

I want a very, very high number to represent my total years of experience, and—as a bonus—I get to live those years as an eighteen-year-old. Put more simply, you cannot escape aging, but nobody can force you to be mature! View the world through your inner girl's eyes.

What kind of power do we bring to the sisterhood when we meet and greet our older sisters not as old women diminished in physical strength but as their inner girls? First, the playing field is leveled when our conversations are between our equally young, vital inner girls. Second, our lives are enriched by adding together the great wealth of our years of experience while our inner girls empower us to step to the front and be seen.

If I do not "see" Phyllis as part of my landscape because I am afraid to see women twenty years my senior, how on earth can I tap into the extra twenty years of knowledge she has amassed? If she in turn shuns those ten to twenty years her senior, how much will the depth of her work suffer?

We all have a very strong tendency to confine our interactions to those within our biological age group. This self-imposed restriction is usually counterproductive. When I first saw the thirty-five-year-old woman at the conference, my immediate thought was that this beautiful young woman had better things to do than talk with me. Maybe she did, but when I asked her a question, our years were not an issue. She responded to me as a contemporary and I to her. The same was true of my interaction with Phyllis. I knew she was an integral part of the conference and, as such, powerful. Why would she want to engage in conversation with me? Again, by stepping out of my age group, I found another "sister" who indeed was my contemporary.

Is it possible that our inner girls should be representing us to the public? I am delighted when younger women consider me part of the fun, and I adore those older women who bring along their own inner girls. We all learn from one another, and that in the end is our goal. We gain intimacy, support, and empathy, but even better, this genuine appreciation for our close emotional ages opens the door for a lightness of spirit that can only be described as play.

Can you indeed play your way to a fuller life? Absolutely!

Laughing Out Loud

The Red Hat Society is an evolving group of second-fifty-year women who quintessentially are showing the vengeance side of aging! Their hallmark is wearing purple clothing with red hats and accessories. They give their inner girls free rein, and they play simply because they can. Groups are forming spontaneously, playing with the journey into their second fifty years. At last count, membership numbered 150,000 and growing. (See the appendix to find out more.)

If you live in the Southeast, you may have heard of the Sweet Potato Queens. Their credo states that a southern girl will do anything for a tiara. What fun! Over 1,900 chapters of women are now taking their inner girls out to play as they laugh in the face of the aging process. (See the appendix for more information.)

To some, these groups may appear to be an overreaction. Our mothers did not behave this way. Well, it's not too late for them! Our mothers and grandmothers are joining the play too. The invitation to all second-fifty-year women stands: call upon your inner girl to guide your way, and play your way into a wonderful old age.

The psychological effect of laughter and play is healthy. Joking and laughing are integral to how the human mind processes and allows us to accept the unacceptable realities of life. Much in life is beyond our control. Jokes put a fence around these uncontrollable events and help us cope and feel safe again. Jokes let us accept the unknown and support our ability to grasp and categorize sad events as bearable. Traumatic events must be categorized as acceptable to ensure our sanity. Joking and laughter are the psychological equivalent of receiving a blood transfusion when we are in danger of bleeding out. We do not forget the pain of a particular day, indeed we can easily reenter the horror or sorrow we felt all over again, but with laughter we validate our right to survive and we go on. Humor brings relief from our inability to change a story that is out of our control. Joking and laughing empower. Tap into them!

What can you do to understand the power of your second fifty years? Where can this play lead?

All New Playmates

Openly engaging in conversations and establishing relation-ships with older women provides an even greater gift, as the following story illustrates. Several years ago, I met an energetic woman at a retirement community in Hood River, Oregon. I assumed she was visiting a relative and struck up a conversa-tion. She told me that she ran the small convenience store and led the calisthenics on campus. I expressed surprise that she lived there at her young age and asked if she was married to an older man. She responded that not only did she live there but, at ninety-four years of age, she was the oldest resident. She in-stantly became my idea of what being ninety-four could be. Because of her, my internal map now has a perfect picture of what I can be at ninety-four, both physically and emotionally.

Whom do you want to be like in each of the decades ahead of you? Think of a fabulous woman you know in each age group who can be your role model, both visually and emo-tionally. Write a name in each of the following blanks to cre-ate your own team of more life-experienced women:

This woman is my picture of what I can be

at 60-plus _____

at 65-plus _____

at 70-plus _____

at 75-plus _____

at 80-plus _____

at 85-plus _____

at 90-plus _____

at 95-plus _____

at 100-plus _____

You may be thinking at this point, I have all the examples I need within my own family circle. You are welcome to fill in the lines with the names of family members whom you adore. But please go one step further and find some new "old" friends. These can be current acquaintances. Just take the relationship up to the next level. They may be neighbors or fellow church or club members that you can invite into your personal circle. Your new friends will have new stories to share with you. You will be amazed and inspired.

Moving beyond Family

Another good reason to add new old friends to your group rather than just family members is that your relationships with your family members in general and your mother in particular are psychologically loaded on two levels: (1) your sense of adulthood and (2) your sense of mortality.

Your Sense of Adulthood

To better understand familial lines of authority, think back to your high school friends who were a year or two ahead of you in school. They held positions of authority then and they still do. When I was a freshman, my best friend, Chic, was a junior and her sister, Judy, a senior. When we get together, even thirty and forty years later, those positions still hold. (Of course, I now make the most of being the youngest!) I still feel a quiet unspoken respect for their authority, even though we are only a couple of years apart in age.

On the other hand, I have a new friend Judy's age whom I consider my contemporary, not my senior. You see, when we make a new friend, our relationship is a blank slate despite any age difference. We start a new friendship as equals and we get to be as grown-up or as "grown-down" as our new friend. All expectations are established within the framework of that particular friendship.

As you add new older women to your list of friends, you will be amazed to find these new old friends dare you to explore flights of fancy you would never imagine trying with your younger friends or even with older family members. Hearing fresh ideas, finding perfect acceptance, sharing secrets, talking inner girl to inner girl—that kind of closeness is the goal!

Trading Moms

With your family members, you feel an even deeper implicit, if not explicit, line of authority than with your high school friends. Although no one may love you and adore you and think you are as perfect as your own family does, families still have acknowledged positions of power and respect, particularly mothers and daughters.

The mother-daughter relationship can be fabulous or not. What never goes away is that Mom is Mom. Her role has, out of necessity, been very directive. It has been her responsibility to teach you how to cross a road as a child and live through disappointing romances as a young girl. How many times have you turned back into your twelve-year-old self in her presence?

Mom may not intend it to be this way, but somehow you slip from adult-adult into adult-child authority patterns. I am often confused by my own adult daughter's need for my approval, and I have to question whether I am as guiltless of judging her as I assume myself to be. We have to accept that moms trigger emotional reactions whether they intend to or not.

You can be fabulous friends with other women your mom's age because they are not emotionally vested in your personal choices. They see you as an equal. On a certain level, this could be considered trading moms. "Traded" daughters get all the value of "Mom's" added experience without those pesky emotional triggers.

If your mother reads this book, she may be more ready to agree with this idea than you expect. You may be surprised to find that your mother already has friends that are your age.

Don't give up on being a grown-up with your mom. Be amazed at the relief from childhood patterns you experience in your relationships with other older women. Then light-heartedly leave the door open to being a better friend with your own mom. Trading moms and daughters may be the gateway to a more equal relationship with each other.

Mortality versus Immortality

Although having equal power in a close friendship is important for your inner girl, of deeper significance is your sense of mortality, or rather immortality. This is the second reason to add nonfamilial older women to your list of role models. Remember when as a child you had parents, grandparents, and even great-grandparents still living? In the natural order of things, these people represented wonderful protective layers between you and death. Now, as your older relatives reach the end of their lives, you miss those you have loved and depended on, but something else has also happened. Your protection has disappeared. You are moved one level higher in your family hierarchy. You are one step closer to becoming the final protective layer for the next generations of your family. Death is psychologically frightening and your inner girl is very reluctant to agree that your life will someday end. Your natural desire is to be young and live forever.

At my family's first reunion held after my Grandma Tessie's death, my eldest aunt had become the matriarch of the family and we all gathered to enjoy seeing one another again. I was shocked to see that all Tessie's great-grandchildren were becoming young adults. When did that happen? I realized I had moved up a layer in what I perceived as "the family onion." As a child, I was the core, protected in successive layers by parents, grandparents, and even great-grandparents. As time passed, I bore children and my great-grandparents died. I was no longer at the core of the family. Events had pushed me into a higher ring. At this reunion, I realized that only one layer—my parents—stood between me and the outside layer of my family. I am fortunate to still have both parents living, but a day will come when I will be called with the rest of my generation to spend the duration of my life as the ultimate protector of my progeny. I will answer the call because it is the natural order of life, but I will seek support from my older and more experienced friends.

Friendships with older women partially fill the void left by the death of beloved family members and are their own reward. Yes, these older friends will also die eventually. Because you love them, you will miss them horribly, but their deaths do not affect your sense of mortality or increase your generational responsibility the way losing a family member does. Remembering the enrichment they have brought to your life is a great source of strength in your grief.

Seniors Rule

Now that we love and listen to our inner girls, we have one more enormous task ahead—getting the word "senior" back. The word should mean that we have earned a special honor and reward for persevering. There is historical precedent.

Remember as a freshman in high school how it felt if a *senior* asked you to the prom? Then you spent three long years earning that senior status yourself. You got to spend a whole year in that awesome position, and graduation was simply the best. What power you had!

Going to college was fun, but you were a freshman, looking up one more time to the seniors. This time you were lucky if it took only three years to reach senior status. But yes, that was where the power lay. Once again, you graduated.

In the business world, the title "Senior" is also a reward. You must work hard to become a vice president and even harder to prove you deserve to be "Senior Vice President." Do you shun the title when it's offered? Absolutely not. "Senior" means power. "Senior" confers authority!

Now you are a senior once again—this time for the rest of your life. You are ready to enjoy the power, and what do you find? Not only is there no party, there is instead a quiet shame.

Being a senior is not a disease. Do not shun your journey toward old age. Accept that great age brings a certain physical decline. Refuse to define your elders by what they can no longer do but rather by what they are still doing. With all your potential and sense of inner girl, work to dispel the shame and bring back the honor of being experienced.

As baby boomers enter their second fifty years, it is their responsibility as a group to reestablish the value of this position.

In doing so, we owe enormous recognition to the generations ahead of us who have so valiantly put up with our shenanigans.

If seniorhood is a dark room, then it is our responsibility to turn on the lights. Currently, fifty-three million women are over the age of forty-five, and only AARP seems willing to publicly claim an interest in our demographic.[2] Where is our voice?

Shifting appropriate respect to the over-fifty crowd will take no less fomentation than women's suffrage in the 1920s or the Black Power movement of the 1970s. Senior power must begin among seniors. Power is *taken* by a group, not *given* to it. One woman asking to vote was not heard; millions of voices were. Change must come as a united voice from within our own ranks and it starts with the understanding that senior is an *earned* status.

It is time for a change. *We* must remove the shame attached to the aging process within our own ranks. We must subscribe to the beauty of a long life. Plan to be part of the change. Honor those ahead of you because it is their turn. When you honor the inner girl of all second-fifty-year women, you and they will regain and retain power.

Second-fifty-year women unite! If we do it right, we can joyfully proclaim, once again, *Seniors Rule*.

Chapter 3

Starting on the Inside: Developing a Passion for Your Future

*T*housands of pioneers crossed the Rocky Mountains following the Oregon Trail into Idaho and on to Oregon. They did this in the face of great hardship and with no particular promise of reward. Hope drove them. You have probably read books or seen movies about pioneering, whether about prairie life or the westward migration. You cannot begin to appreciate the full impact of those stories, however, until you actually travel a good portion of the trail yourself, if not by wagon train, then at least by car.

When you travel west across the prairies, it comes as a complete shock that the Rocky Mountains do not ascend gradually out of the prairie but rather rise precipitously, thousands of feet in the air, abruptly ahead of you. Some pioneers chose to spend the rest of their lives staring up at but not traveling over those formidable crags. For them, staying on the prairie represented giving up the dream, the potential, and the experience.

What does this have to do with your second fifty years? If you let the prairies of Missouri, Nebraska, and Wyoming represent your first fifty years, the journey across these prairies has been treacherous enough for any thrill seeker. Along the way you hear about menopause but have no idea how rudely it looms ahead of you.

Trepidation about this part of your journey and the enormously changed landscape of your second fifty years is a logical response. The difference between you and the pioneers is you have no choice but to go forward into the unknown. However, there is good news! You are not the first to make the journey. Thankfully, there is a path that can lead you to magnificent heights. The breathtaking vistas from the top of the mountain can only be imagined from the bottom.

Asking the Way

If every pioneer had walked alone, each looking for a personal route over the summit, far fewer of his or her descendants would be here to tell the story. Instead, the pioneers asked directions and then followed in the steps of those who had successfully crossed ahead of them.

Women often complain that men tend to wander until they find their destination rather than ask directions. As you reach your second fifty years, you may not be much better. You probably hear friends your age ponder the best route to a full life. Or you may watch Goldie Hawn and Susan Sarandon discuss life's purpose with Oprah. Their conversation is interesting, even enlightening, but none of them are over fifty-six years old. They can recount their experiences so far, but they lack pertinent information that comes only with experience. Where are the voices of those age seventy-six or ninety-six to speak about the shortest, safest route to a fulfilling life?

You cannot ask your contemporaries for answers because they are only as knowledgeable and experienced as you are! To ignore available knowledge gained by those ahead of you is a foolish waste of resources.

Increased Awareness

Are you smarter now than you were fifteen years ago? You should be *much* smarter. Pretend a friend fifteen years your junior were to ask, "What do you know now that you didn't know at my age?" What would you tell her about the importance of self and the importance of relationships? Give yourself credit for the knowledge you've gained and your more enlightened values. On the other hand, if you feel you have learned little, there is still time to grow. Those who do not grow are doomed to a sad, regret-filled old age.

As you age, your body may go downhill, but your experience and knowledge go uphill. The value of your increased awareness far outweighs the physical changes you experience. You indeed are well repaid for the loss of your youth. Do you want to be only as smart as you were at thirty (which was much smarter than you were at twenty)? Absolutely not! Does it not follow that someone ten to twenty years your senior has knowledge you don't? Might she help you avoid those dead ends you will trek into if you insist on trying to find your way without help? You will go further and easier, and therefore have more choices, if you ask directions. If you want to find the smoothest, grandest, most awe-inspiring trail to the top, just ask!

It All Starts with You!

You can ask directions from those with more experience, but you must understand your core self before you can apply those lessons. Ask yourself: Who am I? Why am I? How do I fit into the whole scheme of my universe and at what cost? Where do I end and where do you start? Questions like these form the basis of your emotional development from birth to death. Revisit them now to clarify who you are and who you wish to be for your second fifty years. Some days you will feel comfortable with your answers. At other times you'll feel frustrated by what you don't know. Throughout life the beauty of knowledge and the discomfort of the unknown go hand in hand. Just when you have mastered one life skill, another becomes necessary. Just when you seem to be in control, your plans fall apart. Your knowledge is always insufficient. The unknown keeps jumping into the mix. This unknown factor can be the result of nature's whim (it rains on your garden wedding). It can be the result of political forces (the wrong governor gets elected). It can be caused by deficiencies in your support system (your best friend is out of the country when your dog dies). It is often, sadly, caused by your family (your mother questions your judgment one time too many). The greatest unknown of all is the story of your journey from birth to death.

Maturity means allowing for the unexpected. Life is a series of problem-solving events, some large, some small. Think about it: if you ever lived a single day that went exactly as you planned, with no adjustments, you would mark that day on your calendar and celebrate its anniversary every year.

If your plan for the day is a straight path, the adjustments you make throughout the day are forks in that path that you are forced to take. Only at the end of the day can you look back and know where you've been. You make many of these adjustments to your original plan instantly and you do not count them as disappointments. Other decisions require serious diversions from your desired destination. These hard choices require an expenditure of emotional energy, and your reaction to this expenditure depends on your force. Does dealing with the unexpected throw you into a spiral of negativity or have you allowed room to formulate positive solutions to your dilemmas? Do you wallow in a problem or move on to the resolution? Your spirit, your willingness to move on throughout this process, showcases your strength. Energy, force, and strength: these are the ingredients of a well-lived life.

There is nothing like your second fifty years to put a major fork in your path. Did you ever dream you'd be this old, let alone stay old for the duration? Following this new path will call on all your resources.

Your life is your responsibility. Your answers to who? why? how? and where? represent the paths chosen on your personal journey to either a life well lived or opportunities lost. When you seek answers from those more experienced than you, they happily provide signposts across the unknown landscape. Their knowledge can smooth your journey.

Choose to passionately continue the journey. This is a one-way path after all! How far can you go?

The Aging Dilemma

Do not hide from the facts. Do not deny reality. You have problems to solve now that your younger self didn't have.

Surprisingly, the one serious universal problem with aging is neither disease nor poor health. Many people live into their nineties and beyond in great health. The big problem is that just when you have reached a point where you have great knowledge, fabulous experiences, and quite a few answers, you tend to disappear. Aging is almost like being erased. First, your hair starts to lose its color and your skin loses its vibrancy. Then, thanks to the effects of gravity, you lose height, your shoulders round, and your stature shortens. In time, your step slows and your energy flags. Just when you have achieved exceptional life experience and knowledge, you are overlooked and ignored in the rush of life. You simply do not command the presence of youth.

You have two options: allow the decline or fight back. If you and your inner girl choose to fight back, you can easily regain your presence and power through the way you dress. An inner girl loves color and has fun with style. You also regain your presence and power with your inner girl attitude and sense of humor. Fight to replace what nature has taken away from you. Now you are aging with a vengeance!

You must *be seen*. This is not an egotistical goal because you must be acknowledged before you can make a difference. And you and your inner girl are meant to influence the world around you.

If you are just entering your second fifty years, the time ahead potentially represents over fifty percent of your life. It will certainly contain all of your experience, all of your understanding, all of your passion, and all of your talents. You would not turn back even if given the opportunity. Embrace your age within your particular stage of life. A better understanding of your processes and those of your older sisters will enrich your journey forward because in the end, your goal is to become very, very old—healthy but old.

There is power to be shared between those ahead and those behind. What a concept—empowered women honoring empowered women of all ages.

So, Sis, pull on your comfy sweats and curl up in your favorite chair. Let's look at how we got to this point. Let's note where we currently stand. Most importantly, let's set our sights on where we want to be.

This is no small goal in our constantly shifting physical and emotional environment. We gain strength from the insight of the sisterhood and we know this secret: these are not "little old ladies" but simply girlfriends. They, like girlfriends everywhere, are here to love and support us through the unknown. They just happen to know more!

Walk through the portal to self-understanding about your ages and your personal stages to another of the most universal truths of your second fifty years: age is a leveling agent.

Age, the Great Leveler

You may be groaning that the loss of your youthful advantage is exactly why you are less than enthused about the road ahead. You mourn the loss of your young beauty, rightfully so. But beauty has many faces. You are able to create and define beauty if you so choose. That is part of the irreverence of the second fifty years. If there are many forms of beauty, then aging is one of the greatest!

If the types of physical attractiveness during your teen years and early adulthood were lined up on a seesaw, it might look like the illustration at the top of the next page.

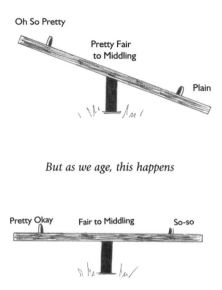

Oh So Pretty

Pretty Fair
to Middling

Plain

But as we age, this happens

Pretty Okay   Fair to Middling   So-so

With age, the distance between great beauty and complete plainness is greatly shortened. In fact, competition has nearly disappeared! Both extremes, great beauty and utter plainness, have been eliminated.

While the woman who was a great beauty in her thirties is mourning her loss of presence, more average women in their middle years find their voices and their faces. Have you changed? Yes. Will you change again? If you are lucky. Long life hands you repeated opportunities to revisit your assets, strategize the best expenditure of your talents, and execute your positive plan to reach the next stage.

Stop trying to "find" yourself. Finding oneself is for young adults. It has to do with the need to separate from your parents' identity and establish your own world-view. Instead, begin creating and recreating yourself in your second fifty years. Tools for creating yourself are the gifts you will open in chapters ahead. Inner girls love gifts, especially the gift of beauty.

From Absolute Beauty to True Beauty

Absolute beauty is a relative and transitory beauty. It is found in abundance in the young but is an entirely foolish gauge for one's whole life. True beauty, on the other hand, is available to everyone. True beauty happens at every age and at every stage of life.

This new definition of beauty looks ahead, not behind. Beauty at fifty is different from beauty at thirty. Seventy is beautiful in still another way. True beauty cannot be fully achieved until you stop using the unique beauty of youth as the only definition of beauty.

Claim your own beauty and it is truly beautiful. Step out of the wallow about what is not and into the energy of what is. Beauty is where you find it, how you define it, and what you make of it. It may be a soft beauty or a gentle beauty, but it deserves to be appreciated. If you lived the life of a wallflower in your youth, you no longer have an excuse to merely *watch* center stage. Now, grab your inner girl and *be on* center stage. A magical secret from the sisterhood is self-invention.

Barbara Walters was interviewing beautiful young stars shortly after the movie *10* was released. She asked Bo Derek and Cheryl Ladd if they considered themselves to be tens. Both women demurred and said they were only eights or nines. When Barbara asked her last interviewee, Bette Midler, if she were a ten, Bette looked at Barbara and asked, "You mean on a scale of one to ten?" When Barbara said yes, Bette responded, "I'm at least a fifty-five."[1] How quickly Bette showed the one-to-ten scale to be deficient.

Not everyone is an absolute beauty, but everyone can be a true beauty. Bette is a true fifty-five. So are you if you claim to be. Who you are is who you are. That is your beauty. Start with that and, as you continue to read, you will find wonderful secrets that let you adjust your attitudes, increase your power, and keep you excited about life—the life you are living now and the life you are planning to live into the far, far future.

This stage of life is your personal reward for living this long. Many have not been privileged to journey this far. It is indeed a great gift, becoming older.

Embracing Fifty-Plus

A mother turning fifty was asked by her thirty-year-old daughter if she was depressed about getting so old. The mother wisely replied, "Not at all. It is the alternative that is depressing!"

Live by the motto "Better over the hill than under it!" Celebrate! Dare to try new things and make waves. Wear more color and bolder accessories. Take up a sport. Learn to play the piano. Take singing lessons. Get comfortable with your reality because you are strong and, yes, beautiful. You deserve to stand out.

This is your time to be powerful in your own sphere and make a difference in your own way. Encourage and empower those around you to step out of the shadow and be seen. When you encourage others to shine, you move forward into greater and greater power. The second fifty years is already your best fifty years because it is what you have.

You have the opportunity to create exactly who you want to be. You are free to define your own beauty and to acknowledge and tap into the power of the sisterhood.

Put your options to the test. Since your choice is either to live or to not live, choose not only to live but to live it up!

When You Are over the Hill, You Pick Up Speed

On the twenty-first anniversary of my eighteenth birthday, I threw a little surprise party for myself. I rounded up ten of my closest friends and took them to a local flea market where I turned them loose with this directive: "You have one hour to find me a present and a way to wrap it, all for under $1.00."

At the end of the hour, we piled back into my Chevy Blazer and drove to a local pie house for lunch and to open my "presents." Although several of my friends were experienced flea market shoppers, my favorite gift was a cup purchased "as is" for twenty-five cents by an absolutely overwhelmed first-timer. In big red letters it stated, "When You Are Over the Hill, You Pick Up Speed." The sentiment was cute enough, but the physical condition of the cup was of greater interest. It was missing its handle and exhibited multiple chips in its glossy enamel. The cup looked as if it had rolled down the very hill it described. Why would anyone have saved this cup for resale?

To this day, after nearly thirty-seven anniversaries of my eighteenth birthday, this cup graces my desk as a pencil holder. I love the story of how I received it and I love the oh-so-true sentiment. Life truly does go faster and faster. These are great years, even for all the wear and tear!

Faster Is Better

Have you ever met people who love living so much that they seem to change the world just by walking through it? One attitude defines them—they expect to take charge of what they can affect and also expect to let go of what is beyond their control. This attitude moves mountains—at least little ones. This attitude alone sets them apart. This attitude is powerful.

Have an attitude about the years ahead. Affect what you can; let go of what you can't. Promise to yourself that you will use attitude to make your way to the top of the hill, the front of the line, or anywhere else you are needed.

Imagine life as a roller coaster ride. When does the fun really begin? Is it the slow white-knuckle crawl to the top of the hill? No! It is the rest of the ride. Where do you find the most excitement and the best view? In the front row. Honor your inner girl and grab that seat.

How do you maximize the feeling of joy in the journey? Let go of your fear, raise your arms over your head, and yell "Woo-hoo!" Try it! The rush of positive feeling is immediate.

When you are over the hill, you pick up speed. Woo-hoo!

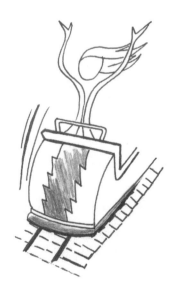

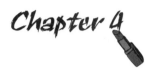

Chapter 4

Strategic Planning:
It's Not Just for Business

Strategic? The word itself sounds like work. Actually, it is just a $100 word that means that you operate by design to thwart a potential enemy. Strategic planning entails putting yourself in the most advantageous position before engaging the unknown. For our purposes, it represents your ability to artfully prepare for your second fifty years. Tips for strategizing will be offered throughout this book. This chapter does not provide answers but rather a framework for personalizing your own goals as you progress through the book. You have done strategic planning in some form many times in your life. Getting acquainted with the formula for successful design is just a precursor to living your life with great purpose and passion.

Step back in time to when you were a young child. Remember how adults leaned intently toward you with the query, "What do you want to be when you grow up?" This inquiry started at a very young age. Surprisingly, you had a ready answer—teacher, dancer, nurse, cowgirl, or some other romantic profession that had caught your current fancy.

Years later, as you worked your way through high school, the question became, "What are you going to do when you graduate?" You may have planned to get married, get a job, or go on to college. You were expected to have a focus or plan for what came next.

If you went on to college, you now had to declare a major. Were you premed, prelaw, education, or maybe business administration? You could not graduate without following a prescribed curriculum.

Then you wanted to start a business. To be successful, you had to have not just a plan but a "strategic" plan. Unlike school, your course to success was not set out for you. You had to make up the whole thing. It was advisable to look for mentors (wise teachers or coaches) experienced in your line of business and ask their advice. You did not want to "reinvent the wheel" when there were shortcuts to success. You were no fool, so you asked for advice.

You may be one of those who knew early on exactly what you wanted to be and indeed fulfilled that early vision. Being a wife and mother may have been part of your plan. More than likely, your interests went through many phases even as you entered adulthood. Nonetheless, you had a dream of becoming someone who fulfilled some mission and was accomplished in your field.

Near the end of the first fifty years, another word becomes central—"retirement." Successful retirement results from once again working from a plan. Your plan addresses how far into the future you will need funds and how and where you will physically live. But have you planned for your psychological needs? Do you retire and stop living? Do you retire and stop contributing to the world around you? The simple answer is "maybe." What is your plan?

"Spending" Your Life

Sound business principles can also assure profound living. Creating something unique and filling a need with your life is your business. You are a niche business. Only you can bring your personal skills and experience into play.

Business runs on wealth called "capital." Likewise, your life is your human capital, much like money in the bank. Your allotted years represent your living allowance put on automatic withdrawal. You cannot invest your years to make them increase. You cannot save them for another day. You can only spend them. You spend them each day, one moment at a time, until one day the account is empty.

How valuable are your second fifty years? How valuable is planning your spending? How critical are your decisions? Only you can decide.

Most readers of this book have either fulfilled or frittered away their potential for their first fifty years. The challenge now is to plan for the second fifty years. You have been so busy getting an education, raising a family, and running a business that you have done little to this point to address how you will spend the rest of your life. You have heard the term "misspent youth." How much worse is it to misspend your second fifty years? Do you have a plan in place to become 65, 75, 85, 95, and yes, 105? Will you *let* your second fifty years happen or *make* them happen? Do you ignore the future or anticipate the future? There is no power in denying the process. There is, however, untold power in embracing your potential and planning for every stage ahead.

Mentors

You alone have the power to become a fabulous woman who changes the very face of aging itself. Pick fabulous coaches for the aging process. Find wise teachers to share their life experience. Forestall the misspending of your own life; your capital is too precious. Mentors reduce the mistakes you make and increase the odds you will accomplish your plan. Mentors understand your dilemmas because they have gone before you. Your mentors will bless you with great insight and expectations and help you feel a zest for what is ahead instead of sorrow for what is behind.

As a woman with older friends, you get to be the "youngster." In return, you honor their contributions and inner girls while sharing your energy and vitality. In business, this is called a win-win scenario.

Planned Aging

You can let age happen or you can make it happen, but it will happen, *if you are lucky*. Do not take this journey blindly. There is a huge difference between letting your life happen and making your life happen. Everything you have learned and accomplished in your first fifty years can—if you plan for it—make the second fifty years a true glory.

Build a visual picture of how strong, fun, and full of life you can be at each decade. Using the Florida Keys as a reference, picture each decade as one in a string of small islands or keys.

How many keys are in your chain? Do they teem with life? How would you make each one beautiful? Now build a bridge from one to the next. Emotionally connect your decades in your mind. Realize that the only way to live a long, full, beautiful life is to actually get older, moving to the next key. How many islands and how many bridges do you see? Will you not learn lessons on Key Fifty that will improve the beauty of Key Sixty and every decade after?

Plan to be one of those women with a passionate attitude. When you live a beautiful life you affect the world forever. You, indeed, live forever by making a difference that makes a difference that makes a difference.

How often do you hear or say, "I don't want to get old"? Yes, you do. What you don't want to get is unhealthy. Aging is not a medical condition. Plan to age successfully and healthfully. Healthy old age is a goal that is both to be wished for and attainable. Add one more key to the map of your future.

Don't just plan to get much, much older, but plan to get cuter and cuter! If you age with a vengeance, if you follow your plan, you maintain greater power and control of your own destiny. If you give up your power, you will have nothing to give and you will not make a difference. Indeed, without a plan you will disappear. For help with your plan, consult your inner girl.

Entering a Second Childhood

You have heard talk of a second childhood. Plan to enter your second fifty years not with dread but with a sense of wonder. The hallmark of childhood is curiosity. As a baby, you spent hours observing something as simple as your small fists clenched in front of your face. Plan to carry that innocent wonder and intense observation through your second fifty years. A whole world of experience and knowledge is waiting for you to gain and also waiting for you to share it. The arrogance of the first fifty years assumes that real living ends somewhere slightly past fifty. That's not true—if you have a plan.

Because you now make your choices with adult experience and inner girl exuberance, you can enter not just a second childhood but an informed childhood. Here's where being a little irreverent and unpredictable pays big dividends. Try these ideas:

- Play dress-up with your inner girl.
- Costume yourself for just today.
- Say and do what you want.
- Ignore old admonitions like "you can't," "you shouldn't," or "be quiet."

In this phase, you can be whoever you wish, on purpose. Remember, for the second fifty years, rules are only suggestions. Now is the time to honor your emotional age before your chronological age. Define your own way. Be able to say, "This is who I am. I am not here to be voted correct. I am not here for you to decide what I should and shouldn't do."

You finally have permission to present yourself and your inner girl as you wish. It is vital at this stage to know exactly the "you" that you want to present to the world. Who do you want to become as you progress? Do you want to become a "sweet little old lady" or a "grande dame?" Put it in your plan.

Plan to truly love yourself as an individual. Believe in your right to be different. Let go of false perfection as defined by others, including your mother or Madison Avenue. You are perfectly imperfect, a one-of-a-kind masterpiece. Be at least a fifty-five on a scale of one to ten!

Living well does not happen at random. Living well is the result of developing a set of skills and attitudes that maximizes your personal interactions, minimizes your disappointments, and validates your value. Living well means that you age with style, panache, and yes, high energy—in your own way. Plan for it.

Creating the "You" Business

Creating, by definition, requires art, skill, and invention as well as imagination. The business world has honed this creative sequence into definable steps to success. Guess what: put your life in place of the business entity and voilà—success!

The process starts with your vision of the future.

Vision

> In business, vision statements start with the "big picture."
> They address the definition of success many years into the
> future. These big picture statements are then broken into
> five-year plans, ten-year plans, fifteen-year plans, and so on
> to show strategically how success will be won.

Your vision is your purposeful mental image of something not visibly apparent or yet come to pass. It is your imagined success of future events. Having a "vision" is not some new, scary, unknown concept. You have used it many times in your life. You had a vision of graduation from school that you worked toward. You had a vision of your wedding day that you planned for. Any success you have experienced in your life to date has followed your first having a vision. How much more important is having a vision of your second fifty years, not only the full fifty years but in five- and ten-year increments?

For example, take the statement "I plan to live to be 120, then get shot by a jealous wife." If this is part of your vision statement, then you show that you expect to be strong, funny, and yes, desirable far into future. You plan to be someone whom people will notice.

Refer back to chapter 2, page 32 for the five- and ten-year increments you have already established. Why did each of these women make your list? Write a key word or short sentence stating the power each represents to her decade.

_____

_____

_____

_____

_____

_____

Mission

Companies next develop a short two- to three-sentence description of exactly what they hope to achieve. This mission statement shines a light on the special function or duty they hope to fulfill. These few sentences are the compass that points a company straight toward the future. New ideas are tested against the mission statement before being pursued.

Remember the concept of the living eulogy from chapter 1? Here's where you get to apply the principle and develop your own life plan.

You, like a company, can write a few sentences that state your hope for your second fifty years. What would you most like to be said about you in your eulogy? Write that eulogy. When you have a clear picture of the difference you can make in the lives of others, you can plan to do just that.

For example: "_____ was a wonderful woman. Her legacy is the inspiration she gave us to live life out loud. The changes she brought in the lives of those she loved will be passed to future generations. We were never safer than when within the range of her beautiful smile. Her ability to love was unsurpassed. We are incredibly enriched for having known her. The world is made infinitely poorer at her passing."

Take time to write a potential tribute to yourself. Look at your collection of tributes. Use rich expressions gleaned from what has been said about these lives that have already made a lasting impact.

_____

_____

_____

_____

_____

Now post a copy where you can read it daily. Your life will follow this course.

Challenges

Businesses take time to anticipate the roadblocks between them and their final vision. They plan ahead for the extra effort that will be required to surmount difficult issues to reach their goals. Little in business is easy. Looking at, anticipating, and strategizing solutions to potential obstacles heighten a company's chances for success.

What are your challenges to a successful second fifty years? Life is not always easy. Looking at, anticipating, and strategizing answers to your potential issues heighten your chances for a fabulous second fifty years.

Take note of these challenges here. For example: "I will guard my health by staying physically and spiritually active."

_____

_____

_____

_____

Mandate

Some companies include a mandate or authoritative order. They feel "required" to perform their service because of a particularly great need in the business world that is not being met by anyone else.

You, as a unique individual with skills and experiences all your own, may just as easily carry a personal mandate. Some are called to heal. Some are called to teach. Some are called to hold. If you sense a place you "have to be," then you are called. This is your mandate. Only you can fill it, and you must. If you have felt called during your first fifty years, you already have a great start on your plan for your second fifty years. Answer for yourself, "Where am I meant to make a difference?"

_____

_____

_____

_____

_____

_____

Goals

Businesses set both long- and short-term goals to foster the expected outcomes of their vision. This is a very active and ongoing process. Again, goals are necessary steps to successfully fulfilling a business's stated purpose.

Is who you are, the difference you will make, and the legacy you will leave any less important than those of a commercial business? How will you successfully live the next week, year, decade? Will you make life happen or let it happen? Goals make the difference.

Write your goals in this space. For example: "I will be seen, be confident, live long, live well, and make a difference. I will also grow cuter and cuter over time!"

_____

_____

_____

_____

_____

_____

Major Objectives

Objectives are concrete steps to make all the vision, mission, and goal statements actually happen. This is where businesses stop talking about what they will do and take physical action. This is when a business becomes real.

Write your major objectives here. For example: "I will walk thirty minutes a day. I will eat balanced meals with lots of fruits and vegetables. I will volunteer for _____. I will surround myself with people that value me and I them."

_____

_____

_____

_____

_____

_____

Executive Summary

Businesses revisit their plans many times throughout the year. The top executive in a company is responsible for keeping everyone within the organization on target. Frequent summaries of successes and unanticipated challenges provide the most current direction for the organization.

You are your own chief executive officer. Do not waste your second fifty years waiting for someone or something to happen for you. Be in charge. Frequently summarize your successes and weaknesses. Increase your power by being in charge of your own destiny. Power is not given, it is taken. Take your share.

Once your plan is in place, it is still not enough. There is the issue of "image" to address. How do companies position themselves against look-alike businesses? How do they create requests for their product or service? They create a "brand."

Branding

No business thrives without letting the public know what it does differently from all the others. Neither do you.

Your personal brand is the image people have when they think of you. Do you inspire? Do you terrify? Do you disappear? You have a high degree of control over this, especially in your second fifty years. This is where creating yourself becomes imperative.

You are your most important product. You affect the lives of those around you by design or by default, either enriching or impoverishing their world. When you actively work to be a positive influence, you are. When you only wish to influence, never stepping out, you lose effect and the world is a lesser place. Nobody can escape this issue. Choose to influence by design. This is not a difficult step. Something as simple as having a ready smile speaks volumes.

The tools to understanding and presenting your strengths are presented in the following chapters. Do not worry if you feel your brand is weak. The secrets of the sisterhood will provide all the tools you need to find the second fifty years your most powerful and successful. You will create your own vision, your own future, your own brand.

Catherine Kaputa, a personal branding strategist, states, "Self-branding is creating an asset out of who a person is and what they can do. A self-brand is a strong personal identity based on a clear perception about what that person stands for and what sets them apart from all others."[1] She promises that strong emotional bonds are created with one's public when a branded person knows her strengths. She further states, "Successful brands have an irresistible attraction. Brands are in demand. They are people magnets."[2] How important this concept is for your second fifty years.

You have a unique, evolving story. Make it relevant and memorable. Your legacy is not what you want to say but what, in the end, is said about you. Be yourself, but be your best, most aware self. Tell the truth, especially about your strengths. Create your own style—your own brand.

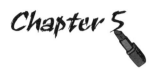

Chapter 5

Self-Love: Making It Unconditional

Self-love, pure and simple, is seldom felt and even less often spoken. Self-loathing, or at least body-part loathing, is a far more universal female behavior. This lesson became clear one day during an interaction with a beautiful ninety-six-year-old customer. She was everything you could hope to be at ninety-six—tall, strong, clear-eyed, and healthy. People were always amazed to find out her actual age.

Her grandson's wedding was in the near future and she needed help finding an appropriate dress. I estimated her size to be a perfect ten. I was rather new in the apparel business and I had purchased a few dresses that were not as friendly a fit as most of my clients needed. One dress in particular required a perfectly proportioned body and good height to carry the look. The color was appropriate for this customer and the style was fashionable enough to qualify for a special event. I selfishly knew that I needed to sell the dress to this woman or I would have it in stock for a very long time. As I matched the dress to my customer in my mind, I said to her, "You have such a perfect figure. I have the perfect dress for you."

She stopped momentarily, placed her hand over her barely rounded abdomen, and said, "Oh, I have a tummy."

Shocked, I responded, "You are kidding, right? You have the stomach a fifteen-year-old would die for." This perfect ninety-six-year-old did not accept herself as perfect. I felt an immediate implication toward my own sense of self. I put my arm around her, looked her in the eye, and asked, "Does this mean we women go to our graves not liking ourselves?"

She responded quietly with a slow nod, "I guess so."

Until that day, I had always assumed that at some magical moment I would be content with who I was and how I was shaped. I thought I would stop picking on myself and concentrating on my "flaws." I assumed I would outgrow unflattering comparisons of myself to that perfect model that exists only in my mind. I thought focusing on my flaws was childish, and I presumed that when I "grew up" I would stop being so cruel to myself.

That evening I went home, looked into the mirror, and kissed the fantasy of regaining my twenty-year-old body good-bye. I knew I wanted to live long enough to become like my beautiful, healthy, ninety-six-year-old customer. I also knew that on some absolute level, at age forty-three, I was prettier and certainly stronger than I would be at age ninety-six. If I expected to live that long, I needed to start loving myself just the way I was today from now forward, whatever my age. I determined that day to begin enjoying each year of my journey toward ninety-six as being the very best year of my life.

How do you determine for yourself that you are living the best year of your life? It may take a little attitude adjustment.

Wasted Years

Have you noticed how the wish to look younger is a wish to look the way you did not appreciate at the time? And yet you don't accept the way you look today as perfect either. If you waste your forties grieving over the loss of your twenties, what do you gain? I had already wasted my twenties and thirties not feeling perfect enough. At forty-three, I stopped wasting my life grieving over the years behind me and instead began to honor my journey toward a wonderful old age. The gift of accepting myself as perfect came none too soon because menopause was nipping at my heels and I was about to be truly tested in my ability to love myself.

Picture Perfect

Has this happened to you? You smile for the camera and when the photos come back, some older, rounder woman has replaced you in the shot? Few second-fifty-year women love their pictures at the time they are taken. If you don't destroy the photos, put them aside for a few years, and then revisit them, what happens? You probably wonder, "What was I thinking? I looked pretty good!" To resolve this dilemma, when you have your picture taken, immediately tuck away the photos for a few years. Then when you take them out, you will be pleased with your appearance! This experiment proves that you have been a beauty for the whole journey. There is just a short time lag in your realization. Work to apply your self-loving sense of beauty to today's reality.

How do you balance your internal wish to meet an acceptable standard with the reality of your personal gifts? With self-love. A personal assessment of your own value is not open to public vote. Self-love says, "This is what I have to offer and it is unique."

Your task is not to change your weight, your exercise program, or your hair color. Your one responsibility is to accept yourself—as you are today—as completely fabulous. That is not to say you will not change your weight, exercise pattern, or hair color later, but change based on loathing oneself is transitory while change based on loving oneself is permanent.

This chapter charts a path only you can take. No one can do it for you. Someone telling you what to believe about yourself won't change your life. There is no magic here, but if something rings true, make it part of your belief system and magic will occur.

Repairing the Damage

It is never easy deciding to love yourself. You were born with a sense that you were perfect, but it has been chipped away since early childhood. The process may have started with parents who showed you less than unconditional love. It may have been continued by other children being cruel at play. These early experiences are programmed into your subconscious. Like old continuous-playing eight-track tapes, they never end. Negative comments replay in your mind whenever you feel judged. It becomes natural to adversely compare yourself to someone you consider physically closer to perfection than you. This habit is the result of trying to fit yourself into someone else's mold rather than accepting the unique package that is you.

You deserve to be seen as the individual that you are. There is only one you. The package of traits you have to offer is unique. Think about it. How rare and valuable is an original painting by Picasso or by Matisse? Although each artist used a completely different style for completely different tastes, works by both are still extremely valuable. You may prefer one style of art, but that does not diminish the value of the other. Likewise, you have your own style, and you do not have to be loved universally to be loved deeply. Appreciate your place in the human spectrum as a unique work of art. Surround yourself with those who appreciate your style. You are what you are, and that is more than enough!

Barbie Programming

Other factors besides childhood memories contribute to the negative tapes that play in your mind. One of the biggest influences for baby boomer women is the Barbie doll. With her well-developed figure, she was a far cry from the Betsy Wetsy baby dolls of the same era. You may not have consciously expected to grow up to look like Barbie, but subconsciously you were programmed to believe that you would eventually have large firm breasts, a small waist, and long shapely legs.

Barbie's figure was "normalized" in 1998 by decreasing her bust and increasing her hips. Still, what is the reality of Barbie's proportions today? If Barbie were the five-foot-four-inch height of the average American woman, she would measure 31-14-26. Her legs would require a 32-inch inseam versus the 27-inch average, and her feet would be five inches long. Although Barbie's proportions are an impossible model of beauty, unloading years of her imprint is no small task.

Once you arrived at puberty, you could read supposedly appropriate teen magazines like *Seventeen*. There you were exposed to girls your age that never had acne, weight issues, or weird hair days. As a result, your subconscious believed that the images you wished to emulate should be attainable. Did your mirror ever agree?

As a college coed and young adult woman, you were then exposed to more Barbie-like images in magazines like *Cosmopolitan*. Perfectly shaped women were presented, not in their natural state, but in an airbrushed, chiseled perfection beyond even their actual beauty.

Fairly new to the market is the magazine *More*. It is meant to support perimenopausal and menopausal women through this confusing stage. However, the magazine is full of models again picked to show a form that most of us did not have twenty years ago, let alone today. An article about an older woman may feature Raquel Welch or Lauren Hutton, who are in their late fifties to early sixties. Beautiful women forty years ago, they are still beautiful women today. You may love to see how well they are doing, but do you need to have their natural and/or enhanced beauty as your standard?

From girlhood on, women are constantly exposed to an idealized vision of the female form that rarely occurs in nature. Even those women one might judge to be near perfection are often uncomfortable with their ability to meet their own self-imposed perfect ideal.

Return to Nature

What can you do in the face of these "too perfect to believe" images? Simply step back into nature where there are innumerable images of beauty, not just one. See yourself against the greater beauty of the whole natural world and suddenly your place in it becomes clear. You are meant to fill a spot as beautifully as every other creature and every botanical wonder in our world.

Horse Sense

Here is how I learned this lesson. From the age of six, I lived and breathed horses. I had a whole library of horse books and regularly studied the "horse" entry in the *World Book Encyclopedia*. The walls of my room were covered in horse posters, and my favorite magazine was *Western Horseman*. I didn't spend much time playing with dolls, but as I went through puberty, it became apparent even to me that I was "flawed" when compared to Barbie. My chest was too flat and my hips too wide. I was uncomfortable, concerned that I was somehow unacceptable. I thought about my dilemma. How could I categorize myself as acceptable?

Then it occurred to me that horses come in many shapes and sizes and every breed has different strengths, temperaments, and performance abilities.

All the beautiful models in *Seventeen* were like Thoroughbreds—tall, fine-boned, fast, and high-spirited. This visual ideal was only one proportion, one physical type out of many. What if every horse in the world was a Thoroughbred? We would be missing so much.

I knew I was proportionately no Thoroughbred, but a lot of other horses had characteristics that might match mine. I realized, given my build, that I most resembled my personal favorite, the nimble quarter horse. Quarter horses have strong hindquarters and are shorter and meatier than the Thorough-bred. They are sprinters and have high endurance and even temperaments. They are beautiful in their own right. The fact that I had a different shape did not preclude my being defined as beautiful.

If you study the horse kingdom, you too may find a breed that describes you. Think of the Shetland pony, the cutest of which are the miniatures. Short is beautiful. On the other end of the scale, people drive from miles around to see the fabulous Budweiser Clydesdales. They are amazing and powerful horses. Bigger is beautiful too!

Can either of these breeds aspire to be Thoroughbreds? Can the Shetland grow taller? Should the Clydesdale lose half its weight? Of course not. Why would they even want to? Their beauty stands alone. So does yours. If you are a Thorough-bred, lucky you. If you are another breed, lucky you too. The animal kingdom is designed to provide great diversity in sizes and shapes of beauty. Redefine your personal standard and love the diversity you see around you. Adore the Thorough-breds and respect their qualities, but honor and love the Clydesdales too!

Maybe you know nothing of horses. This same exercise works with dogs. You may not be a greyhound, but who cares? What about cats? If you haven't explored the new breeds in this category in recent years, you are in for a wonderful surprise. There are as many interesting cat types as dog types. The most sought-after new breeds have traits that were formerly considered flaws. There are hairless, bent-eared, curly-haired, and bent-tailed breeds. Do you see? Former "flaws" are now bred *into* the line for their unique beauty.

How much more valuable are your own special traits? How can you showcase them? Embrace the reality of the beauty around you with a self-accepting attitude and you become beautiful.

Totems

One day, a tall, elegant, full-blooded, American Indian customer asked for "anything giraffe." She picked a few items and mentioned that the giraffe was her "totem" because of her height and long neck. Being nearly six feet tall as a teenager in the 1940s, she literally stuck out at a time of life when most of us hoped to blend in. When asked what she meant by the word "totem," she explained that in her culture a totem is an animal or object from nature that is meant to represent you and symbolize your sense of self. Her giraffe totem validates her unique traits. With it, she honors her height and her long neck. Her totem shows the world that she perceives herself correctly as impressive and majestically tall.

You too can pick a totem or multiple totems from the animal or plant kingdom, as many as you please. When you define yourself through the beauty of nature that you feel represents you, you introduce yourself to your public as a unique whole woman.

Take time to revisit nature as if you were a curious child. Go to the zoo. Go to a dog show, a cat show, an exotic bird show, a horse show, or a flower show. Or go to the library and get books on these subjects. Revel in the diversity you see. How boring would it be if all horses were Thoroughbreds, all dogs were greyhounds, and all cats were Persians?

Appreciate natural variety, then pick your own totem *in each category*. While you are defining yourself this way, something special happens. You'll see totems that also represent those around you. Some people, you will realize, are giraffes and others gazelles. Some are greyhounds, others pugs. You'll recognize toucans and finches, dahlias and sweet peas. All are magnificent in their own right.

You, my dear, are part of a beautiful, diverse world. There is no one perfect human form any more than there is one perfect flower form or one perfect animal form. You are perfect just the way you are.

Picking Totems

Take time now to determine which species of each group on the list below best represents you. Does this selection come to mind because you are tall or short? Does it represent some unusual physical characteristic? Does it echo your proportions? All the better. Do not skip over or treat this exercise lightly. It may be one of your most valuable tools for true self-appreciation. There are many definitions of beauty. Define yours:

Horse _____

Dog _____

Cat _____

Bird _____

Fish _____

Wild animal _____

Amphibian _____

Flower _____

Tree _____

Do not stop with this list. Look at all of nature as an expression of your unique place in the scheme of the universe. You are meant to be seen. You are meant to make a difference. Do it being just you!

Confidence

Make it your goal to be seen. Being seen takes confidence— lots of confidence. Without confidence, you cannot make a difference. With confidence, the world is yours. How do you gain confidence? How do you know what it looks like? It's easy. Watch confident people.

Confident people are self-defined. They have a firm belief in the value they offer. Confident people appreciate differences in the world around them and do not compare themselves to others. Confidence means you present yourself perfectly as is, and the world agrees.

Do not be confused. Arrogance is false confidence. False confidence is demanding while true confidence is giving. False confidence takes all the attention while true confidence gives undivided attention.

Watch truly confident people and you will see that all their focus is on those around them, not on themselves. They assume they fit in so they are free to pay attention to others. This is not surprising because when you are at your most confident, self-awareness disappears and self-assurance takes over. Confident people are in demand because they take so much interest in others. Confident people make the world a better place.

Do not expect your confidence to be expressed exactly like someone else's. Confidence is more like a perfume. Some wear it lightly, some more strongly. In the same way, people will differ in their response to your confidence. You may be quietly confident and affirm an action or you may be boldly confident and propose the action. Still, you make a difference when you know and acknowledge your worth.

Learned Confidence

If you have never felt truly confident, it is possible to learn. Like any other subject that you master, confidence will take study and practice, but it can be yours. Do not be afraid of confident people. Confidence welcomes confidence. Even the most confident people have bouts of self-doubt, but they surround themselves with positive energy and step back up to the plate.

If you are not naturally confident, you can use a shortcut. Fake it! Pretending to be confident is like using training wheels to get you rolling. It is a simple human truth that behavior precedes belief. If you act as if you are confident, your mind will work to make your action true.

Here is the trick: When you are headed into a situation where you feel less than confident, take a deep breath, close your eyes, and imagine how you would behave if you were feeling perfectly confident. How would you stand, what would you say, how would you smile? In other words, how would you *act* in this ideal world? Actors act; so can you. Walk into the room and pretend. Act exactly as you would if you truly felt confident. When you do, an interesting thing happens: your *act* is perceived and accepted as true by those around you. Soon, you are no longer acting but actually feeling confident.

Do not wait to *feel* confident, just *act* confident. Your sub-conscious will thank you by validating your confidence. You will actually be confident. The process is magic.

Recreational Surgery

Sometimes one physical feature negatively affects your confidence and how you feel about yourself. You may choose to surgically alter an area that seems out of line with the vision you have of yourself. This is not necessary surgery. That is, it is not needed to save your life. It is purely recreational. Cosmetic surgery is not for everyone, but it is a choice to consider.

My personal creed is egocentric, "If I was born when there are plastic surgeons, they must have been put here for me!" Surgery does not stop aging, but if done correctly, it can re-fresh your look.

Before proceeding with cosmetic surgery, consider the fol-lowing: If you opt for surgery, are you going to interfere with that part of you that truly sets you apart? In other words, is your definition of unattractive valid? The first time I saw Barbra Streisand in a movie, I was struck that this star did not have a perfect nose. How dare she? I thought. Didn't she know her nose needed surgery? By the end of the movie, my whole perspective had changed. Barbra was beautiful *because* she had a different nose. Thanks to Barbra, I became a nose connois-seur of sorts and to this day appreciate strong facial features in both men and women. It doesn't matter whether Barbra loved her nose as is or was afraid to risk her voice to change it. I have to say thank you, Barbra Streisand, for your nose.

Another Barbara influenced my thinking. While George H. W. Bush was president, there was some discussion about his wife's prematurely aged appearance. Many said she needed to have facial surgery. Her refusal to do so had me a little confused. Couldn't she see that her husband looked younger than she did and that she should do something about it? It is now many years later and to my knowledge Barbara Bush did not "fix her face" to suit me or anyone else. Over time, her husband, George, has come to look Barbara's age. And Barbara? She has a soft yet powerful, matriarchal, and grandmotherly face—nearly the identical face she had ten years ago. She has stopped aging and is just beautiful. I now appreciate her decision to go natural. So to you too, Barbara Bush, thank you for your face.

I am a great admirer of still another Barbara, Barbara Walters. Barbara appears to have had some recreational surgery. She is stunning. She is my idol of femininity, strength, and brains for someone in her seventies. I love that she appears to have nipped and tucked a little along the way. So thank you too, Barbara Walters, for your face.

So you see, your appearance is a personal journey. Who do you want to be twenty and forty years from now? Cosmetic surgery is not for everyone. You may never consider it. Good for you. On the other hand, you may have a surgery calendar already planned twenty years into the future. Good for you. Do not judge others by their choices and do not be judged as to yours. Everyone's goals are personal. Do you want to become a powerful but sweet-looking grandmother, or do you want to be a grande dame? You get to choose. So do I.

From Ordinary to Extraordinary

More important than making surgical changes is actually taking everything we know about ourselves and making the very best of it. The life of one amazing woman—legendary fashion editor Diana Vreeland—gives us all permission to create our own identity. This story "of a homely, unloved girl who transforms herself into the queen of American style" is excerpted from Eleanor Dwight's biography, *Diana Vreeland*.

[Diana Vreeland] grew up in New York City in the first decades of the twentieth century. She had dark curly hair and dark eyes, and she looked smart and perky, but she didn't have the classic, angelic features and blond curly hair of her little sister, Alexandra, who was four years younger. The obvious differences between the children—in appearance as well as disposition—prompted some bitter remarks from the girls' mother. One day [Diana's mother told] her older daughter, "It's too bad that you have such a beautiful sister and that you are so extremely ugly and so terribly jealous of her. This, of course, is why you are so impossible to deal with." Diana remembered, "I simply walked out of the room. I never bothered to explain that I loved my sister and was more proud of her than anything in the world, that I . . . adored her. . . . Parents, you know, can be *terrible.*"

This poignant reminiscence some seventy-five years later illustrates how Diana came to transcend the pain of her childhood, just as she would later transcend the painful moments of her own career and family life. . . .

When she was fourteen, Diana began a diary that reveals her adolescent angst. She wanted to separate herself from the ugly girl she imagined she was and cultivate a charismatic personality and a distinctive appearance. Her extroverted qualities and her ability to capture people's attention with her smart outfits were a carefully calculated way of expressing her true self. . . . Diana worked hard on enlarging her vocabulary, improving her ice-skating, and her manners. It was only a matter of time before she would become her own most inspiring ideal.

By the time she made her debut in 1922, she was seen as attractive and charming, outgoing and amusing.[1]

Diana went on to refine an innate style that would become distinctively her own. Her personal credo was "to embellish the world and make it more vibrant." She made "a startling first impression wearing bold yet simple clothes. She had a great color sense [and combined] originality and whimsy in using objects as accessories."

At fourteen years of age, Diana unwittingly set in motion a perfect strategic plan with all the elements we discussed in chapter 4. Her vision? To embellish the world and make it more vibrant. Her mission? To cultivate a charismatic personality and a distinctive appearance. Her goal? To be extroverted and express herself with smart outfits. Her objectives? To enlarge her vocabulary and improve her ice-skating and her manners. Did having a plan work for her? Yes. "By the time she made her debut in 1922, she was seen as attractive and charming, outgoing and amusing."

With her confidence in place, Diana was ready to make a positive mark on the world. Her personal style led to a position at *Harper's Bazaar*, where she wrote the column "Why Don't You?" The theme echoed her personal credo. "Don't just be your ordinary dull self—Why Don't You be ingenious and make yourself into something else? [Have] limitless imagination." She challenged readers to "stretch themselves beyond the ordinary."[2]

After twenty-six years at *Harper's Bazaar*, Diana became editor-in-chief of *Vogue*. There she led the vanguard of changing ideas about beauty. "She personally liked the new look because it validated her own atypical physiognomy." Diana found beauty in the unusual.

"Diana Vreeland died on August 2, 1989. Throughout her life, Diana wrote, she had 'always been looking out for girls to idealize because they are things to look up to because they are perfect.' But since she never discovered 'that girl or that woman,' she had done the next best thing: She became her."[3] So can you.

Thank you, Diana, for perfect imperfection. Thank you for fulfilling your vision to embellish the world and make it more vibrant.

So many gifts are contained within these few paragraphs about Diana's life. She epitomized the "be seen" philosophy and she went on to make a better world where women could be perfectly imperfect. She embraced and encouraged an atypical beauty in her magazine. Learn from Diana's life. With no extraordinary physical gifts and in spite of her mother's failures, Diana unconditionally accepted and loved herself. She alone defined her brand and created her legacy: "Why Don't You?"

Unconditional

Unconditional, applied to yourself, is one of the most frightening words in the English language. Unconditional means *absolute*. Unconditional leaves no room for "except."

The tendency to focus on your least favorite features is natural. Do you end your self-assessments with an accepting "Looking good!" or a depreciating "Dang my _____ (breasts, hips, feet, hands, hair, and so on)?" Do you note *your own* least favorite feature, either for better or worse, in others? Your issues are personal. Most of the public is obliviously unaware of them. Women with small breasts who wish they were larger do not understand that a woman with large breasts may wish for smaller ones. You accept her breasts; she accepts yours. How much better if you each accepted your own.

Have you ever received a compliment for a trait you didn't think particularly interesting? Someone once complimented my eyebrows. Until that day, my eyebrows were just eyebrows, but after a discussion about my friend's struggle to shape hers, I consider my eyebrows to be special. A compliment says much about the complimenter, but let it also put your focus on your own strengths.

Never deflect a compliment by mentioning a negative aspect of yourself. One day when a young teenager of my acquaintance had obviously taken pains with her dressing, I mentioned how beautiful she looked. She immediately pointed to her face and said, "I have a pimple."

Until that moment, I had not noticed the pimple. How often do you point out the "pimples" in your appearance? Those around you see the whole picture, not the blemishes. You need to let go of your negative focus. But how?

Make a simple vow to stop picking on yourself—today, now, forever. If Diana Vreeland was perfect, so are you. Changing your mind-set involves getting in touch with your subconscious. If you have spent years listening to and giving your subconscious mind negative cues, feeling negative about yourself is natural. It is now your duty to reprogram your mind to fully accept your personal being as perfect. Nothing anyone else says to you can change the way you think about yourself. Only you can do it.

A simple phrase can become your mantra in times of weakness and self-denigration. The beginning is easy enough: "I love myself." It is the last word of the sentence that may make you sputter: "*unconditionally.*" String the words together and repeat them to yourself whenever you feel emotionally threatened. I love myself *unconditionally.* These four simple words represent possibly the strongest, most healing sentence in the English language.

If you have never had permission to feel this positive about yourself, saying these words may feel self-absorbed. It is not. It is the basis for all healthy relationships in your life. Saying "I love myself, unconditionally" quiets the taunts of cruel voices from your past—whether of parents, schoolyard playmates, a spouse, or yourself.

No one can love you more than you love yourself. If you have low self-love, you have a low capacity to hold the admiration of others. Has anyone ever made a positive difference without first being admired for being something special? No. Being admired is a necessary and healthy goal.

Being special is an unlimited commodity open to all. Accept your own value. You will not believe kind words from others if they are not kind words you have already said to yourself. Surprisingly, you cannot be genuinely kind to others when you are not first genuinely kind to yourself. Practice being kind to yourself daily, hourly. But first be sure that what you expect of yourself is reasonable.

The Importance of Others versus Self

A myth often referred to as the American Dream causes untold damage to people's sense of being successful. This supposed dream states, "You can be anything you want to be if you work hard at it." No, you can't. You can excel only when you honor your natural gifts and natural talents.

John Bradley, president of IDAK Group, has developed a list of fifty-four different human skills.[4] No one excels at all of them, even with training. Few are masters at more than five to nine of these fifty-four skills, and each combination of five to nine skills creates a different strength, called a skill set. You have a highest and best use based on your individual skill set.

Follow your dream to its logical conclusion. If you don't have the voice, give up opera but solo in the choir. If you can't solo in the choir, run the sound booth. Just find where your skills make the most pleasing music. That is the true American Dream. When you passionately take your rightful place in the chain of human interactions, you find joy, peace, excitement, and a full life that indeed makes a difference. You will know you have found your highest and best use when what you do makes your heart sing.

If you have five to nine specific skills and those around you have different combinations of five to nine special skills, how many people does it take to complete the full range of skills necessary to maximize human potential? Enough to hold a party! No one stands alone as special. Rather, each person is special as part of a range of needed talents. You *need* people to be different from you. Other people *need* you to be different from them. How wonderful to celebrate the differences in others while honoring the special talent you bring to the mix. Honor others and expect to be honored in return.

Picture a small basket in your lap and drop a token in the basket for each of your special skills. You have permission to have only one token, but you do not have permission to hide it from view. Your token, your skill, is needed to complete the full potential of humankind. Humans are social or tribal creatures meant to share their abilities.

What would you do if money were no object? What part of your work experience would you have done for free? Analyze these natural pleasure points because they suggest your strongest abilities. Success is its own reward. Find where success and joy meet for you.

Take time to list your talent(s) here. For example: I'm organized. I enjoy meeting new people, I enjoy working alone, I enjoy public speaking, I love to plan events, I love to work with numbers.

_____	_____
_____	_____
_____	_____

Analyze how this list represents the gift you have to contribute. You are here to complete the chain, not be the chain. No one else has exactly your mix of skills and experiences. Assume your rightful place as a one-of-a-kind treasure!

Twenty-one Days to Love

Repeat this simple mantra, "I love myself *unconditionally*," every night as you fall asleep. As you diligently repeat this phrase for twenty-one days, your subconscious will work to make it true. Just three short weeks will undo years of self-loathing and self-depreciation.

Complete self-acceptance—what a promise! You will hold your heart and soul in your own loving hands. You will treat yourself with respect and honor. You will present this unique wonder of nature to those around you. It will be so peaceful, you will never fall into self-loathing again because you have your truth in place: I love myself *unconditionally*.

Of course, there is a counterbalance to loving yourself. The mythical story of Narcissus tells about a young man looking only at his own reflection in a pool, unable to love anyone else. As you work to love yourself unconditionally, you are not wishing to be narcissistically self-focused but to be a complete, loving human being. The necessary balance is found in having *warm regard* toward others.

Chapter 6

Other Love: Offering Warm Regard

*U*ou have learned to say, "I love myself, unconditionally." You know your self-love is in balance when you can add the phrase *"I hold all others in warm regard."* Notice you are not expected to love all others unconditionally. You do not have to agree with everyone, nor should you. Others will not agree with you, nor should they. How do you keep disagreement from being disagreeable? How do you honor people who disagree with you? You live in warm regard.

A better understanding of human nature may make your affirmation of others easier. Loving yourself means you pick your friends and loved ones with great care. According to Dr. Harville Hendrix, author of *Getting the Love You Want*, we scan five thousand faces to pick one we find specifically attractive to us. Other people are also scanning five thousand faces to pick one attractive to them.[1] Therefore, for two people to find each other equally attracted and form a bond takes work! The energy and time required to maintain that bond means that you have time for many more acquaintances than friends and time for more friends than loved ones. In other words, you are selective.

How do you feel warm regard toward those other 4,999 who will never be more than passing acquaintances? Some of them may actually irritate you. You are not expected to find every set of human characteristics charming. Likewise, you cannot expect everyone to find you charming. So you see, there is no time, let alone need, to be all things to all people. You, and everyone around, you must be picky as a matter of efficiency.

The affirmation "I hold all others in warm regard" means people are not required to be anything other than themselves. No one is required to meet another's expectations. You do not expect all others to reach your standards because they are just that, *your* personal requirements. Loving yourself unconditionally means that you accept yourself as unique. Holding all others in warm regard means that you leave room for every other human being to be self-defining also. Your self-regard is in balance.

Viewing the World

Personal views are always narrow because you can know only what you have actually experienced. It is natural that those who are close to you in beliefs and temperament will be your closest friends, but be open to other viewpoints and you will discover new vistas.

Picture four inner girls standing on a summit. One is facing north, one south, one east, and one west. Will their views be identical? Of course not. Should each one argue with the others about whether her view of the world below is the correct one? That would be foolish. If they all want a full experience of the view, each will share her vantage point with the rest, and by participating, each will be enriched. Life is like that—you can see only in one direction based on your experience. That others think and behave differently is to be expected. You learn when you are open to human differences rather than being threatened by these differences.

Warm regard means you feel safe about turning away from or moving toward another, different view. Warm regard toward differences opens your own life to nearly limitless opportunities. You increase your experience by sharing viewpoints with others and seeing the world through another's eyes. Sharing ideas does not necessitate agreement. The zenith of warm regard is agreeing to disagree with someone and being comfortable with that outcome.

Still, you honor yourself by setting limits on your involvement with all other individuals. When you are involved with people in passing, expect the unexpected. Be charmed by human differences. But if someone adds nothing to your existence, smile and move on. Do not judge others. They are allowed to be self-determined within their own sphere just as you are in yours. Warm regard allows you to limit how another affects your life. If someone's belief system or behavior is distasteful to you, you feel no need to change them. You simply move on.

Intimate, personal relationships take more negotiation because you are choosing to love another unconditionally. These relationships should enrich—not scar—your life. You have final authority on who gets your heart. But if humankind comes in so many emotional and psychological varieties, how are you to know where your heart is safe? When you better understand your relation to others, warm regard becomes easier to give. Use this analysis: how full is the glass?

The Half-Full or Half-Empty Glass

You hear the question so often, it is almost trite: do you see the glass as half full or half empty? Nonetheless, reexamine this question for yourself. The answer is part of your self-definition and can explain a lot about why you do or don't enjoy certain people. Seeing the glass as half full is supposed to be the better answer. People with an optimistic outlook appear to outlive those who are more pessimistic. Naturally optimistic people feel smug about their can-do attitude since it is the psychological equivalent of being the teacher's pet. Numerous articles have been written offering tips to pessimists on how they can take steps to be more positive. Are these articles ever written by pessimists?

I am hardwired, so to speak, to be optimistic. I worry about virtually nothing. I am stoic in the face of hard truths. I see the silver lining in every dark cloud and believe the best is in store despite the danger lurking ahead. There is actually a psychological term for this condition—"hyperthymia." On some level, this is a dysfunction, but no one wants to "fix" it. I did not get this way by working at it. It is my natural comfort zone, my natural brain chemistry. I would, given a chance, dump the contents of the half-full glass into a smaller glass and end the discussion with, "See, the glass is actually full!"

But what about those who see the glass as half empty? As an observer, I wonder: Are we all hardwired for a reason? Could there be a purpose for seeing the glass as half empty? The universe as a whole is composed of a balance between positive and negative. There is a north *and* a south pole. There are positive *and* negative ions. These are necessary elements for our very existence. Nobody says, "Let's get the negative ions into therapy and change their charge." Is it not probable that there is just as great a need for humanity to have a mix of energies to maximize human potential?

Brain studies show a genetic link to pessimism. If you are hardwired to be pessimistic (negatively charged), it follows that there is a need for pessimism. If you are hardwired for optimism (positively charged), it is because there is also a need for optimism. You have a natural state somewhere on the continuum from optimistic to neutral to pessimistic.

Of course, you move up and move down the scale at times, but you have a basic position to which you default as a matter of comfort. Do not try to be other than you are because you will fail. Changing your intrinsic energy may not even be possible. Accepting and understanding your intrinsic energy is tantamount to establishing deep personal relationships.

Which Type Are You?

In analyzing your position on the optimism/pessimism scale, use the observations below *without judgment* for both are valid world-views. You may hold some characteristics from either side. Check all that apply to you on the list below:

<u>Optimists (+)</u>	<u>Pessimists (−)</u>
❏ are amused by human differences	❏ are annoyed by human differences
❏ turn mountains into molehills	❏ turn molehills into mountains
❏ believe in the best	❏ expect the worst
❏ underreact to actual slights	❏ overreact to perceived slights
❏ are drained by pessimists	❏ are frustrated by optimists

How many checkmarks are in each column? Write the numbers here: + _____, – _____. Now on the drawing below, starting in the middle of the glass, at the water level, circle that number of energy signs on the scale. For example, if you checked two items in the Optimists column, circle two plus signs.

Next, draw a line just above your highest circled sign and another line under your lowest circled sign. These marks on the scale represent your natural comfort range. Likewise, your happiest, best, easiest, most comfortable relations will most likely be with those individuals whose scores fall within this range. You see the world with the same degree of intensity. But also, now that you understand the dynamics 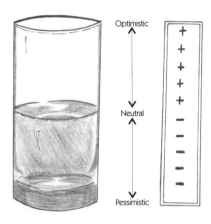 you'll realize that some of your most stimulating, exhausting, and passionate friendships will fall outside your range.

Use this assessment to open dialogue with your family and friends. It is not uncommon to have a blind spot about your actual position on the scale. When you unconditionally accept yourself, you will be open to others' comments about your position. You may become aware that you are giving people the wrong impression. There is no benefit to over- or underestimating your degree of optimism/pessimism because all positions are correct.

What did you learn about yourself from this exercise? What did you learn about your friends and family? Are your marks all above the center line, all below the line, or clustered around the line? Honor your position as necessary to the whole organism of human existence. There is neither shame nor glory in any one position nor is there one best way to view the world. Optimism does not trump pessimism. If you are a particularly pessimistic person, say so and be so.

Pessimism Has Purpose

To an optimist, a pessimist may appear to have an undercurrent of anger or impatience, but usually pessimists are just aware of multiple stimuli. It seems that pessimists are called to experience life so intensely that they have a tendency toward melancholy. Pessimists often use these deep feelings to create great works of art, literature, and music. Because they feel so deeply, pessimists can describe life in ways that optimists may recognize but don't fully appreciate until they see them through the pessimist's art.

Optimists appear to skip lightly along while pessimists map the hills and valleys of human existence. Nuance is the pessimists' arena. While optimists tend to move quickly from one event to the next, pessimists are left, reeling in frustration, to put these events in perspective.

Scientific reports show that those who live in positive energy live longer, healthier lives probably because of reduced stress hormones. But are optimists happier? Maybe if a negative energy position were more acceptable, the stress hormone for pessimists would decrease. Paradoxically, some people are just happier being unhappy. Being told you need to change something that is actually your gift to humanity is not good for the soul. Those who carry negative energy for the human race are to be respected and acknowledged. That is warm regard.

Pessimists unite! You are gifted, not cursed. Or maybe your curse is a gift. Either way, the world is a better place with you in it. You do not need to see the glass as half full. Doing that would destroy the very purpose you were given to fulfill. Pessimism deserves respect alongside, if not above, optimism because pessimists are required to carry a heavier emotional load.

Energy Test

If you are still not sure which kind of energy you have, try these two quick tests:

1. You have just come home from a large party that included many people you did not know before tonight. Question: Are you energized and excited or completely exhausted?

If you are full of energy, you are probably an optimist. Because optimists comfortably skim their environment, they tend to gain rather than expend energy in gatherings. If you tend toward exhaustion, you are probably more pessimistic. Pessimists often tire in social situations because they are more likely to plumb each interaction to its depth, depleting their energy stores.

2. While reading this chapter, do you translate the word "pessimist" to mean "realist"?

If yes, you are a pessimist. While optimists cheerfully believe in a great outcome, and somehow make sweet lemonade from the tartest lemons, you accept the lemon for what it is.

Know Your Energy

Are you Positive Polly or Negative Nellie? Both types make a huge impact in their own sphere. Both are necessary. Both make clear contributions to society. Be clear about what kind of energy you have and with what type of person you prefer to spend time.

In the second fifty years you must be you and you alone. Be honest about where your comfort lies. This analysis does not mean pointing fingers in judgment. There is no better or worse answer; just be true to yourself. Only when you are honest with yourself do you discover your strengths as well as your weaknesses.

Analyze yourself and your closest relationships. Optimists want to fix pessimists, and pessimists want optimists to be more realistic. Is the glass half full or is the glass half empty? Understanding that extreme differences in outlook are not wrong allows for wonderful, nonjudgmental, warm regard.

Intimate relationships are easiest when you pick people within your own energy range. In other words, positive energy feeds positive energy and negative energy feeds negative energy. Unless both people understand and honor their differences, mixing a positive-energy individual with a negative-energy individual can leave them both unfulfilled, exhausted, and confused.

If you are strongly positive energy, don't attempt to fix negative-energy individuals to suit your comfort zone. Pick friends who increase rather than drain your energy. In other words, run with your own kind.

If you are strongly negative energy, don't attempt to make those with more positive energy see "reality." Pick friends who understand and increase your energy. By all means, run with your own kind.

Building Relationships

Assuming you are emotionally healthy, set one goal: to surround yourself with people who let you feel good about yourself. If you happen to love seeing the glass as half empty, do not be shamed into trying to see it as half full. If you happen to love seeing the glass as half full, do not be shamed into seeing it as half empty. People who want you to change to gain their personal approval must be set aside. Pick friends who neither dominate you nor allow you to dominate the relationship. Healthy relationships are based on sharing power but never giving up power.

When you become aware of how your energy plays against another's, you drive confusion out of the relationship. Base your friendships on the energy spent and the energy gained from them. Allow unbalanced relationships to end, not with acrimony but always with your warm regard. Warm regard is your gift to someone you cannot love.

Family Love

Warm regard is one matter with strangers and acquaintances but something else again where family is concerned. Awareness of your natural energy compared to that of those around you is so central to your second fifty years that you should give careful consideration to the individuals in your family that have influenced and still influence your life. From grandparents to parents to siblings to spouse, who around you sees life in negative terms? In positive terms? Define your familial patterns as they exist now. Do your most exhausting and tor-turous family relationships result because of differing energy centers? Give a measure of respect, as you are able, to those most difficult relationships. The deeper your understanding of your personal dynamics within your family, the more re-spect you can give.

True Love

Family relations can be difficult but your *chosen* relationships do not have to be, in fact *should not be*, hard work. A great chosen relationship is your safe place. Getting along with the rest of the world takes work. Your safe relationships let you be exactly who you are. Out of the millions of people in the world, you only have time in your short life span for relatively few true friends. Do not waste your precious energy on dead-end relationships.

Instead, choose relationships based first on shared energy. Then overlay other important interests. Your closest friend-ships should always be with those who understand you. They accept your individuality and everything that makes you dif-ferent. You can trust their acceptance. Who you are is enough for them. You fit together because love is a two-way street.

Disease

What about low self-esteem, depression, or name-calling? Do not confuse low self-esteem and natural negative energy. You may project a false negative energy because your sense of self was denied to you as a child by your parents or as an adult by your spouse. You must spend time finding your true energy. It is possible that you are naturally positive. On the other hand, you may be someone forced to smile at all costs and appear positive when your calling is to pessimism. Move to and honor your natural energy. Where do you naturally rest when you're not filtering your personality to meet someone else's expectations?

Do not confuse depression with pessimism, although they can go hand in hand. Living with depression is not the same as living in negative energy. If depression occurs, wonderful advances in brain chemistry pharmacology can balance missing chemicals. Be sensitive enough to know if your energy has shifted to real depression. The *PDR Encyclopedia of Medicine* offers the following signs that could signal cause for concern:[2]

- Depressed mood most of the day, nearly every day
- Loss of interest in pleasurable activities
- Significant weight loss or gain
- Disturbed sleep
- Constant fidgeting or a slowdown in movement
- Fatigue, loss of energy
- Feelings of guilt, worthlessness, hopelessness
- Difficulty thinking or concentrating
- Indecisiveness
- Recurrent thoughts of suicide

If you are experiencing a combination of these signs, go posthaste to your doctor. Because of changing hormones, depression can increase in your second fifty years. Be in tune with your natural energy state and know when to ask for assistance.

In the end, it is your personal duty to be self-defined. Judging others for the sake of name-calling is childish and has no place in your sphere. Others may attempt to judge you, but only you can accept those judgments. Put those around you on notice: "This is me, deal with it. I do not judge you, and I will not be judged by you. You are safe with me. I need to be safe with you."

Beating Putdowns

What should you do when someone goes on the attack? How do you deal with a gossip? How can you best defuse negative comments? For instance, you might hear someone say, "Susan has absolutely no sense of style." What is the perfect retort? Just agree. Say, "You are absolutely right." Then add the magic words, "and *that's what I love about her!*" The conversation will be over. Try it: "That's what I love about her!" Experience the power of feeling warm regard.

If you are the brunt of a personal attack, again, just agree. For instance, suppose someone you love is angry and says, "You are a total jerk." Answer vehemently, "I am too!" The expected answer, "I am not," only leads to more argument. Agreement ends the confrontation. This tactic is not always easy, but it is always effective.

Puzzle Masters

Relationships are puzzling and it is your job to find where you fit in the picture of humanity. Imagine a puzzle box containing fifteen hundred unique shapes, one of which is you. As a separate piece in the box, you brush against many others. As the picture comes together, each piece has one and only one position to hold. Only a few of the fifteen hundred pieces are meant to fit with you. Those not directly in contact with you hold special places also, but you are not meant to be "close" to these pieces. Find your special position in life's puzzle and allow others to do the same. You are neither superior nor inferior. That is warm regard.

Because you don't get to pick them, relationships with your family will always take a little extra patience. Interestingly enough, being part of a family does not mean members have their puzzle pieces on the same area of the board. Often extra work is needed to maintain these relationships. That is warm regard.

Return to this chapter whenever you feel sad, confused, threatened, or overwhelmed by a relationship. Find yourself and seek balance.

Your Personal Creed

Now that you know your own energy, fill in the blank below. If you need a gentle reminder to balance self-love, other-love, and warm regard, copy this creed and post it where you can easily refresh your conscious as well as subconscious mind.

> I live in _____ energy. I am responsible for the gifts this energy brings. I will not be judged. I will not judge. I will surround myself with people who allow me to maximize my gifts and my energy. I will return the favor.
>
> I know myself. I love myself *unconditionally* and hold all others in warm regard, always.

Part 11
<u>Seen:</u> Your Outside Story

*W*ho you are starts on the inside as addressed in part 1. How you *present* this self-vision is all on the outside. This section addresses how you are *seen* and offers tips and tricks to physically express yourself in the most flattering light.

Learn to be selective, looking for details that will make your look yours alone. Be recognizable for something special. At a minimum, find a "grace note" or two for your look. In music, grace notes, unnecessary to the melody, are added for ornamentation. Pick a personal touch or two and create a note all your own.

Your look is your signature. It signs your personality the way your name signs a letter. Have fun with the process of creating this look whether you make changes in baby steps or quantum leaps. Or make no changes at all. You decide.

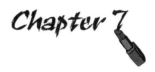

Chapter 7

The Science of Shopping

*B*efore we plunge into the fun of costuming yourself, let's address the guilt sometimes associated with shopping. We'll start with the seemingly incongruous question, why do women outlive men?

The playful answer? Because we shop!

As a personal shopper and image consultant to hundreds of women over the past decade, I often have customers ask, "Why do I want something new when my closet is already full?" Never one to leave a question unanswered, I respond, "Because shopping is good medicine. Something new feels good and it is a lot less expensive than going to the doctor. Plus, it lasts longer!"

What started as a joke turns out to have a basis in fact. Studies of our physiological reactions to shopping show that it is indeed medicinal. You have heard of endorphins, those wonderful hormones that give you such a sense of well-being. They not only make you feel good, they relieve pain and help the immune system fight against invading bacteria and viruses. Most women experience all these benefits from getting something new. The story for men is slightly different.

Why He Doesn't Understand

Have you ever been confused by the male reaction to shopping? It seems as if men think clothing is just to keep people from going naked. Their body chemistry responds accordingly. A program, *Buyology*, aired on The Learning Channel and addressed this specific issue.[1]

A young man of thirty was directed to purchase one pure white T-shirt for himself and a toy truck for his young son. He was connected to sensors that monitored his blood pressure and stress level while he shopped.

This seemingly innocuous excursion provoked decidedly negative physiological reactions in the subject. His systolic blood pressure climbed to 160 and the amount of cortisol in his blood skyrocketed. His stress hormones were at the level of a fighter pilot engaged in actual combat or a riot policeman facing a mob. In other words, shopping caused the same response as going to war and facing real life-and-death danger. He felt no pleasure. Eight hours later, his cortisol level was still elevated. His body was recovering slowly from the "danger" of shopping. Does it now make more sense that the man you love runs into the store, grabs the first thing he sees, and makes a quick exit (if he shops at all)?

It turns out that women shop as gatherers while men shop as hunters. Those times your man gets upset about your shopping may be grounded in an ancient urge to save you from a terrible fate. It is possible that he may be trying to protect you from the horror he experiences. Men, in general, do not understand the thrill that you get when you find the perfect outfit. For him, shopping is warfare. For you, shopping is good medicine.

In all fairness, some men love to shop, and they probably get a positive hormonal response from it. Some women hate to shop, possibly because their systems punish rather than reward the process.

Here's a question to ponder: is it possible that we shorten the lives of our men by insisting that they make personal, time-consuming, heartfelt gift selections for us on every occasion from Valentine's Day to Christmas?

Helping Him Understand

Your man may better understand and accept the importance of your shopping experience if you equate it to hunting for game or preparing for some other favorite weekend adventure.

For instance, on the morning of the hunt, men start early, dress for the occasion in camouflage clothing, and drive long distances to spend hours in uncomfortable surroundings for the opportunity to *maybe* bag their game. The preparation, journey, camaraderie, and stories all have as much significance as the actual kill.

When a woman shops, a more gentle form of these hunting skills is brought into play. Finding the one item that finishes her look is as great a triumph to her as bagging the most illusive game is for a hunter. Like the hunter's, her journey and experience are often as important as the actual buy.

But the evidence in favor of shopping gets even better. In July 2002, The *Wall Street Journal* featured "Keep Your Brain Young," authored by two of medicine's most prestigious practitioners, Guy McKhann, M.D., professor of neurology and director of the Zanvyl Kreiger Mind/Brain Institute at Johns Hopkins, and Marilyn Albert, Ph.D., professor of neurology and psychiatry and director of gerontology research at Harvard.[2] According to the article, genes, proper medical care, and luck all play critical roles in one's health. You increase the odds of staying well by not smoking, eating fatty foods, or drinking heavily and by taking supplements, like vitamin E, daily. But "Keep Your Brain Young" mentions three other factors characterizing those who avoid serious disease and recover better from illness:

- They are more mentally active.
- They are more physically active.
- They continue to maintain a sense of control over their lives.

Indeed, Drs. McKhann and Albert hypothesize, while acknowledging a lack of proof, that one reason women live longer and are healthier than men may be because they shop more: "While shopping they are physically active . . . they are mentally active, comparing prices and making choices."[3]

I Don't Need a Thing So Why Do I Want Something New?

Not only is shopping good medicine, but wearing something new really does make you feel great. You aren't just imagining it. When you wear a new outfit, you have an extra twinkle in your eye, your step seems lighter, and you actually stand a little taller. When you feel good, people notice. Having a new outfit, feeling good, and receiving compliments are undeniably linked.

What about the closet full of clothes you already own? You need to make room for new looks so how do you choose what stays and what goes?

Start with that "perfectly good" suit in your closet that just never gets invited out to play. You may even feel a little guilty passing it over again and again, but in your heart you know it will never make you feel good to wear it. In your mind, this suit has "worn out."

In years past, clothing literally wore out and had to be replaced on a regular basis. Today's modern fabrics are often made with fibers that do not physically show wear even after years of service. So what happens? You become tired of certain items and seldom put them on or don't feel good when wearing them. You may feel dowdy today in something you absolutely loved a short time ago. If so, this garment has run its course. If you haven't comfortably worn an item in the past year, it is probably time to consider sending it into retirement, clearing it out of your closet to make room for outfits you truly do love to wear.

But what if you still can't give your retired garments away? What if you're through wearing an item but you still want to keep it? Quite likely, it means that you are a clothing collector. Don't feel guilty. It is okay to have a few garments hanging in your closet that you never wear. No one ever tells stamp collectors that they must use their stamp collections to send mail across town. You have every right to enjoy the special memories associated with certain items as part of your collection. Your closet should hold both the items you truly love to wear and also a few items you just enjoy owning.

Charity, Not Guilt

If you feel guilty about buying new clothes, have you ever considered the charitable side of buying and then recycling your clothing? I owe this idea to the genius of Lois Harvey, a long-time client. Well spoken and gentle, Lois is not afraid to spend money to feel good in clothes that fit her well and bring her compliments. At one point, I asked her how she could wear everything that she purchased, let alone find room in her closet. She shared the most wonderful secret—her personal, three-way charitable event.

First, Lois, without complaining, explained that concentrating on putting herself together dulled pain she experienced from a chronic health issue. Her days were more physically comfortable because she bought clothes for their medicinal benefit, the good feelings they brought her. Second, she told me she felt that spending money with my small company meant a great deal to the company's fiscal health. (She was completely right about that!) Finally, after wearing her items two or three times she would have them cleaned and donate them, like new, to a charity that did not resell the clothing but gave the items free of charge to deserving women in need. These women now had fabulous "new" outfits that brought them compliments and that magic endorphin surge. What logic. Lois cared for herself, for a small business, and for her needy sisters all with the same dollar!

Like Lois, we all need something new now and again. Spend time understanding your own needs where your closet is concerned. Own what you love as long as you love it, but pass everything else on to those who can enjoy it in your place. If your dog had more pups than you could handle, you would find good homes for them. Do the same with your wardrobe.

Make a clean sweep of your closet. You will be refreshed.

Understanding Your Look

Now that you know the rhythm of shopping and have scientific validation for what you love to do, it is time to start on a journey of self-determination that will let you stand alone as a unique individual in all creation. Your look is not dependent on anyone else but you. The next chapters will guide you through fun exercises and show you insights gained from my wonderful customers.

Understanding your look doesn't just mean buying something new. It also means knowing which clothes you already own are perfect for you so you can wear them often. Having the perfect clothes for you will give you confidence. When you are confident that you have picked exactly the right look for your personality and body type, you literally shine. People listen and talk to you differently.

Learn to create your own way to "be seen" as you continue to read. When you put your look together on purpose, confidence will become your very best friend and follow you everywhere.

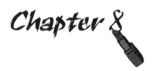

Chapter 8

Playing Dress-Up:
What You See Is What You Get

Do you love to shop? Do you hate to shop? Either way, laws against public nudity as well as your personal modesty mean you are forced to dress. Since you cannot escape making dressing decisions, learn to make more informed, more relaxed choices.

If you take no pleasure in putting your look together, the following sections are designed to put a playful spin on the adventure of defining the easiest, most uncomplicated look for you. On the other hand, if you have always had fun inventing and reinventing your look, you will find dressing nuggets here to add to your personal sense of style adventure.

Costuming

It helps to think of dressing as costuming. The events of your day determine what "costume" you choose to wear. You may be planning to work, exercise, garden, golf, go to church, or just lounge around the house. Have you ever worn your gardening clothes to church or vice versa? Why not? Whether you're interested in the mechanics of putting your own look together or not, you still make rational daily decisions on what to wear. Clothes matter. Learn how to use them to your advantage.

Image

If there was ever a time in your life when your image mattered, it is today. Second-fifty-year women must fight to hold their position. If we age too gracefully, we will go unnoticed in our youth-absorbed culture. Youth—however important—is not the only important segment of life. Yes, it is their time to be young. We had our time to be young—and oh, the stories we could tell—but it is now our time to be older. How can the young wish to live long lives if they see that we do not make a wonderful old age our goal? It will soon enough be their turn to be old. What lessons are we teaching them about the rewards and joys of a long life? We cannot take our image as second-fifty-year women for granted. If we allow ourselves to disappear, the young will continue to believe that one's value ends with the end of one's youth.

In social interactions, it is easier to disappear than to be seen. You have no more than ten to fifteen seconds to visually "say" who you are. It is normal human behavior to evaluate others and be evaluated in very short order based on one's "look." Individual presentation is often more influential than what you have to say. Indeed, many interactions are totally nonverbal.

The next time you are in a crowd of strangers, take a moment to notice how quickly you assess someone's social status, educational level, and economic background. Right or wrong, you make these judgments based on the person's grooming, dress, and mannerisms. In the same way, you project an image to others, whether you wish to or not.

How much respect do you want from others? If your appearance indicates you do not think well of yourself, why should others assume that they must? Taking an extra five minutes to put your look together greatly enhances the responses you receive from those around you. Since you are going to make an impression anyway, make a calculated impression, one that will evoke a positive response.

To do this, people-watch again. This time, analyze why you notice certain people and see which ones hold your attention for five seconds, fifteen seconds, or longer. Answer these questions:

- Based on how each looks, what do you assume about people's personalities?
- Would you want to spend time with them? Why or why not?
- Who held your attention the longest and why?
- Are there points of interest you could adopt for your own look?
- Do you see image-defeating mannerisms, such as slouching, that you are ready to drop?
- What does confidence look like?
- What statements are people making about their vision of themselves?
- More importantly, what statement do you want to make?
- How do you want your ten to fifteen seconds to speak of you?

Punctuation

Your greatest impact comes from your physical presentation and carriage. Projecting a strong but approachable, self-affirming attitude enhances your impact. If how you look and move is your statement, then your attitude is the punctuation to your statement. Is your presentation ended with a succinct period, an open-ended comma, a big question mark, or an exclamation mark? You get to choose. Which of these attitudes do you project?

- ❏ This is me. Period.
- ❏ I'm open,
- ❏ I'm clueless. Does it show?
- ❏ It's all a party to me!

Circle the most appropriate choice for you:

My statement now ends with a   . , ? !
I want my statement to end with a   . , ? !

Better Shopping

If you hate to shop, it may be because you feel overwhelmed by the choices and leave the store feeling sensory overload. If you love to shop, you may have trouble telling yourself when to quit, causing serious damage to your finances. There are two steps to having consistent shopping pleasure and finding the right items for your look: first budget, then hunt.

Budget

Step one is to learn one great word—"budget." Do you have one? No matter how rich or poor you are, a clothing budget is imperative for making your best purchasing decisions. Whether you can afford $20 per month or $2,000 per month is immaterial. Whatever you can afford needs to be spent in a judicious manner. A $20 budget can go surprisingly far. A $2,000 budget may need to be refocused on quality rather than quantity.

Treasure Hunt

Once you know your budget, the second step is to hunt. The trick to buying exactly the right item is rather beautiful in its simplicity. Here it is: Do not walk into a store expecting to buy bags and bags of clothing. Instead, walk in with the stated purpose of buying the one most beautiful item in the store. This provides focus and turns your shopping experience into a treasure hunt.

If you need to build a basic wardrobe, the "item" may be a whole outfit that includes three color-coordinated items of clothing and matching accessories. Once your basics are in place, you will learn to find mix-and-match pieces to extend your wardrobe.

To get the greatest punch for your dollar, choose timeless garments. "Timeless" does not mean boring. Ralph Lauren defines a timeless item as something so extraordinary that you want to wear it again and again.[1] How many shopping mistakes would you make if you always looked for the extraordinary? Almost none.

The Fun Closet

Do you see the potential for playful dressing in this message? By building a wardrobe of safe basics, then spicing up your choices with a few timeless treasures, you will be on your way to a closet that will make dressing fun. Now, what to do with these beautiful clothes?

Dressing the Artist

Since you start out each morning naked, consider yourself a blank canvas. What is your mood today? How do you want to be perceived—as playful, sophisticated, stern, silly? Choose who you want to be just for today! Make your ten-second interactions powerful. Have a message to send and send it well.

Because your dressing decisions project your personality, be a diamond among women. Think about it: diamonds are judged by their carat, cut, and clarity. Let your look project your personality as huge, brilliant, and clear!

Your choices in color, style, and texture help you be seen, be strong, and yes, even be powerful. Think of your life as a movie and design the costumes for your part. Or think of yourself as the wall of an art gallery. Either way, go for rave reviews. Give your public something to talk about!

If for some reason you feel unworthy to be seen, take a moment to look at the mathematical probability that you were even born. Your genetic code and thus your existence could occur at only one given point in history. Yet you are here. Millions of other genetic packages were denied expression on the day you were conceived, not to mention the days preceding and following that day. The fact you are here is an event to be celebrated every day of your life. Cheer! Don't hesitate to be seen!

Choices

You must have confidence in what you love. Do not be afraid to mimic what has worked for you in the past. Your confidence in your choices is what people will see. Don't worry about rules. Instead, think about how your style influences others to slow down and give you an extra five seconds of attention.

When you have confidence in your decisions, you can afford to become playful with your look. Plan to add a little irreverence or surprise. Go slightly over the top; do something unexpected. The unexpected always draws comments and, as a bonus, gives others permission to experiment with their look too.

Being playful means you aren't afraid to try something new. It shows that your comfort zone is expanding. You can determine what is right or wrong for you to wear. When you are confident about your choices, you play in your closet as you play with your friends. On occasion, your taste may even be considered a little crazy. Nevertheless, you find joy in beauty and you value your unique contribution to a beauty-filled universe.

When you dress playfully, you are at your best, you are a pure individual. You are dressing as you choose, not as someone else has told you that you should dress. You dress in a way you truly love. You care about yourself, not as a vain, egocentric attention grabber but as a self-aware, self-determined individual making sure you are a part of the party. In a certain sense, you become your own natural Barbie doll to dress up. Barbie has many costumes and so do you. Dress playfully on purpose.

Define Your Style

How do you define your style? Look first at the types of items of which you have multiple pieces. These are your silhouettes. Do you live in mock turtleneck sweaters, vests, tunic tops, hand-knit sweaters, banded knit tops, or pantsuits? Are the fabrics solids, prints, florals, or geometrics? Picture your favorite, most compelling look. You should be getting compliments when you wear it. If not, it probably needs an accessorizing piece to give it extra punch.

Revisit the concept of branding from chapter 4. Developing your brand ensures you are not a copy of anyone else. Successful branding highlights the person you are. When people hear your name, their mental image of you should be vivid.

There is great power in branding. Forget about being generic. Don't be a car, be a Mercedes. Don't be a vase, be Waterford crystal. Don't be a suit, be a Chanel.

Your style is not determined just by what you like. To a great extent, style is determined by what you don't like. Be aware of colors, cuts, and textures that make you uneasy. If you have made poor wardrobe additions, jettison them. You will never learn to love something that makes you uncomfortable. Ask yourself, is this item beautiful? Is it functional for me? If it is neither, let it go.

Live by the motto "I'll decide who I want to be." You may think such a motto is only for the young, but the youth of America have nothing on you when your inner girl gets a hold on your imagination!

Being "In"

Your costuming needs at fifty, at seventy, at ninety, and older are not identical, but they are not as divergent as you might suspect. You take a sense of style through all of your decades. The ninety-year-old ahead of you does not have to wear what you do to be stylish, anymore than you have to look to the twenty-year-old behind you for your sense of fashion. Honoring your personal taste lets you make the right decisions for the way you live now.

So what is "in"? Is fashion the same for everyone? Is it appropriate for everyone? No! For example, I know what I am going to be wearing in the year 2038 when I am ninety years old (and every year between then and now): tunic tops. Since these tops, popular in the 1990s, are already "out," I will need to find a source for them for the next thirty-five years. My personal love of tunics does not mean that I am unaware of current hiphugger and halter-top fashions. Many of us wore the same combination in the late 1960s. If I still had the figure for these clothes, I might try to wear them again, even at my age. (Is it possible we "fluff up" in middle age because nature is attempting to force us to use common sense about what we wear?)

There is a certain unfairness about what happens to be in or out of fashion at any given time. Take the tunic top, for instance—it is nothing more than a sportier, friendlier version of a blazer. Blazers are basics, never in and never out, so why not tunic tops? Fashions may come and go, but we need our basics!

So, you agree that basics are important, but what about fashion? You do not honor your age by giving up and giving in to a youth-absorbed culture. You honor your age by staying alert to how today's fashions can look great on you. Luckily, you are living at a time when individuality and imagination are expected.

Search out fashion and style appropriate for your age. Capris and three-quarter sleeves, for example, are current fashion trends that should be basic choices for second-fifty-year women not just now but far into the future. Look at what is current and then interpret it to enhance your figure. Honor yourself by dressing to look your best. Your choice of fabrics, accessories, and colors can show your joy in new fashions, but your style must respect your physical reality.

On the other hand, be careful about aging too gracefully. If aging with grace means going quietly, thus disappearing as many do, then plan to age with a vengeance. Acknowledge for yourself that every age has beauty and that fashion and style are life-affirming rituals for a lifetime.

Setting Trends

The sisterhood of second-fifty-year women, as a group, can and should set trends. The media may not listen to one or two of us, but a vocal group gets press coverage. If the sisterhood has to redefine style to be part of the modern scene, then so be it. The way we act powerful, look powerful, and sound powerful has never been more important. This is not a time to be less involved with our position but more involved. Fight age-ism on every level. Compliment shopkeepers on carrying items that work for you and ask for things you cannot find.

The goal is to be an effective sister, a charismatic sister, and yes, a noisy sister! Inner girls unite. If you are tired of being a footnote to the fashion industry, stand up, speak up, dress up!

Chapter 9

Personal Assessment: Why Blend In When You Can Stand Out?

Are you excited about the way you look? If not, it is time to evaluate why not. Is it possible that you are focusing on the negative rather than what is uniquely, positively you?

Do not mistakenly think absolute perfection is the goal. *Absolute* beauty is a mathematical set of proportions that are very rare in the young, even rarer after fifty. *True* beauty, on the other hand, is attainable by all and at every age. True beauty is the total of your physical characteristics and your heartfelt interactions. There is no beauty in isolation. Beauty must be recognized first by the beauty herself, then by her public. In other words, you become beautiful because you say you are!

You are what you are today. You are as strong as you can be today. Your figure is exactly what it is for today. You have assets to be envied and you have challenges that you wish to minimize. You are a complete package of good, bad, and indifferent physical characteristics. Welcome to the human race. Luckily, that package of assets and challenges is all you need to create or recreate your look, your statement, your brand.

Who you are is enough if you *love what you have* and work to maximize your assets.

Since you are in the business of strategizing your second fifty years, then like businesses everywhere you are looking for all the assets you have to build on. It is time to count your physical blessings as well as assess your challenges.

Get something straight right now. *All* figure types are normal and customary. You are not a different size on the top and the bottom. It is the *clothes* that are different sizes. As soon as you see your genetic package as a unique opportunity to stand out, you are ready to love being seen and expect to make a positive impact on society.

Do you have figure *challenges?* Most women do. Do you have figure *flaws?* Absolutely not. Everyone has a "least favorite" body part or two. These body parts may or may not deserve your animosity. In all likelihood, some women would love to have your "problem" in exchange for their own. That being said, most challenges relate to mathematical imbalance.

Rebalance your figure by maximizing your assets while minimizing your challenges. Magically, your look comes into harmony. The goal is to emphasize your proportionate self while minimizing your critical issues.

Assessment One—Your "Best Bits"

Assessment is a way of seeing yourself just as you are today while shining the spotlight on your best features.

Eyes and Smiles

The two most distinguishing features that define you from birth to the grave are your eyes and your smile. Babies instinctively respond to these features. If photos of friends and family revealed only these two features, you would recognize them immediately. No other body parts are so universally recognized.

Given the importance of these human characteristics, *choose clothing and accessories that draw focus to these two features*. In the next few chapters, you will learn how to dress to bring attention back to your face using color, line, and accessories.

This focus on your eyes and your smile doesn't mean you have no opportunity to spotlight other favorite body parts as well. Although you may tend to be self-critical, you need to, even grudgingly, divulge your other favorite "bits." These are the parts that you agree are quite okay if not actually superior to the average. For instance, I list my favorite bits as

Eyes	(wide set)
Eyebrows	(arched)
Smile	(inviting)
Neck	(long)
Hands	(small and slender)
Waist	(small)
Feet	(small)

This list is long enough to show where positive focus should be placed. How do my shopping and dressing decisions differ if I base them on my personal list of "best bits"?

Notice I did not ask you to affirm that my personal list is correct. This list is a personal critique. Until you give yourself permission to have superior bits you cannot appreciate your unique position in society and, in turn, the unique position of those around you. You must love yourself uncritically before you can love another person uncritically. You owe the world that kind of love, but even more, you deserve that kind of love!

The Challenge

Listing your own best bits tends to be a difficult exercise. Listing five to ten *challenges* would be far more comfortable for most women. Few women are willing to admit that even one physical characteristic is okay. How sad that we are so comfortable listing our "flaws" but so hesitant to list our physical assets. Shame on us.

In my seminars, women tend to list positive *personality* traits rather than list *physical* traits. This is not the place to list how "nice" you are. It is time to love your best physical assets and say so. Remember, this is a *personal* critique.

Listing your best bits is the first step toward the physical aspect of branding. It will provide a minimap to focused dressing. Don't be shy. Write your list here.

My Favorite "Best Bits"

_____ _____

_____ _____

_____ _____

Features attract. Make these your featured attractions. You are the star of your own production. You are a whole one-of-a-kind package with many great bits. What's not to love?

What about how you already package yourself? What works and what does not? Can you identify your best looks?

Assessment Two—The Empty Closet

A quick, revealing way to know your favorite look is to answer this question: if all your clothes were stolen, which six items would you truly miss? List them here. Do not rush this exercise. *Feel* your way through your closet.

_____	_____
_____	_____
_____	_____

Do you know yourself better now?

You have gained some physical awareness and some closet awareness. But what about personality?

Assessment Three—Reaching "I Am"

How you relate to the world around you is far more important than any other factor in determining your brand. How are you perceived? How do you *want* to be perceived? Be very clear about who you truly mean to be. There are far too many personality traits to have them all. Be focused.

How do you describe yourself? *Circle as many words as apply in the list on the next page.*

It is normal to feel you possess a little of just about every trait. You do not live in a rigid environment, and you are expected to make adjustments for given situations. Healthy individuals have many behavioral options. But who are you at your core? Who do you most want to be? From all the

I am:

strong	powerful	generous	funny
smart	educated	playful	classy
traveled	kind	confident	interested
caring	curious	irreverent	exciting
positive	giving	foxy	bold
beautiful	humorous	enthusiastic	proud
flamboyant	strong	perky	intelligent
mysterious	dignified	extroverted	introverted

Add a few more terms of your own:

_____   _____

_____   _____

_____   _____

_____   _____

adjectives circled, focus on the six characteristics most important to you. List them here.

_____   _____

_____   _____

_____   _____

Are these characteristics somehow connected with your favorite closet items? You may or may not see an observable pattern yet. You are on a quest to define your personal brand and to send the right signals about it. Plan to hone your traits. Remember Diana Vreeland and her personal credo "Why Don't

You?" You should present your brand so clearly that nobody ever has to guess who you are.

Interestingly enough, once you are clearly presenting who you are, you rise above criticism. In fact, if someone says that you are too much this or too much that, you will know that you have presented exactly whom you want to present. You'll know you no longer blend in.

Think about women who live exaggerated lives—Cher, Dolly Parton, Bette Midler, and Joan Rivers. Their level of definition is hard to top. Understand that you too have permission to be just about anything you want to be. They change for no one and neither should you. Thanks for the great example, girls!

If you are offensive to *everyone*, you have a problem, but if you are offensive to *no one*, you have a bigger problem. Don't play it too safe. Humble acceptance of your own excellence will raise eyebrows. The goal is not to be all things to all people but to be *yourself* with all people. The result will be that some who are wishing for permission to love themselves will move toward you. Those who are afraid to face their inner critics will move away from you.

Remember, you have too many choices in human companionship to deny your true, self-defined personhood in an effort to belong. Be interesting, not bland. Show yourself to be truly outstanding.

How do you use this information to improve the image of your personal brand? How can you learn to focus on your best look? Start with your closet favorites. Your look is often a repeat of items that work for you worn in differing textures and colors.

If you're having trouble finding your best look, maybe your focus is too narrow or maybe too broad. Start educating yourself as to your taste by creating a collage. Have a style journal that you use to jot notes about what you have seen. What felt right about an item for you? Was it the fabric, color, sizing, or cut? Add pictures of interesting clothing from magazines and catalogs. As you continue to collect your favorite looks, you will see a pattern that hints at your emerging style.

Be an observer. Who with your general body type has made a great visual statement? Record in your journal the elements that worked for her. Look around you. People-watching can be entertaining *and* educational.

Assessment Four—Dressed for Living

By now you know your best bits, your favorite wardrobe pieces, and your style direction, but do you balance your wardrobe to match your lifestyle? The final assessment addresses how you actually spend your days. Many women over-buy for one segment of their lives and underbuy for others. How do your dressing needs translate in your own closet? Do you buy a lot of "fancy" clothes even though you spend far more of your week in a casual mode? Do you maybe deny your brand when you are going "just around the neighborhood" or "just to the grocery store"?

Use the chart below to analyze the days per week that you require clothing for different activities. There may be days when you wear all four categories and others when you only wear one category. Now check your closet for corresponding percentages.

	Su	M	T	W	Th	F	S	Total
Exercise								
Casual/comfy								
Business								
Dress-up								

Do you see how the Casual/comfy category is probably a seven-day-a-week need? Be sure that this category echoes your signature look as clearly as the other categories do.

In this chapter, you have explored where you stand today. Love this more defined, wonderful woman. Know that she is amassing tools that will make defining and redefining herself through the years ahead a fabulous, fun-filled project!

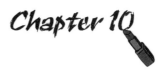

Chapter 10

The Personality of Dressing: Costuming for Your Brand

*L*ife is a stage and you have an act to play. If you so choose, you can project one image now while another image awaits you in the wings. Knowing yourself and a few style tricks lets you create and recreate an interesting human drama. What fun! Give yourself permission not just to play but to play it up! Your life is *your* stage production. Let your inner girl be the director.

You costume each day either on purpose or by default. By your choices, you send a message about your expectations in social interactions. When you develop a purposeful costuming mentality, your look appears effortless and you feel right about it. Now you look confident and expect to be seen. This is no trivial matter. Confidence allows the full expression of your unique beauty and your most engaged interactions with the human race.

But do you always take time to present yourself correctly or only on special occasions? Your daily dress is the basis of your look and how others will perceive you. The young can digress from empowered dressing because their youth alone gives them power. The longer you live, the more important costuming becomes. Dress for yourself first and the confidence that results will let you truly play your way through your second fifty years.

If you have never spent much time putting your look together and feel a little intimidated at your lack of costuming ability, you are not alone. Relax. Branding yourself for your second fifty years doesn't mean you have to look different, just stronger. A few secrets that well-dressed women use, whether by training or instinct, will work just as easily for you. If you have a great dressing instinct, stay with it. If you are shy about your look, a little training will work wonders. Start with who you are, then embellish for emphasis.

Not all looks are good on different *body* types, as you will learn in chapter 12. But did you know that the design of your clothing suggests a personality? In this chapter, we'll see that not all looks are equally good for different *personality* types. As you explore the pages ahead, you will discover how to both pick silhouettes and accessorize for your own personality and lifestyle.

The goal? Be interesting. Dressing style is fluid, not rigid. You may have one best look, but you will learn to add interesting design elements from other styles as accents. Most importantly, you will know exactly what to choose and why you chose it. Knowledge builds confidence.

You probably have a default zone in which you dress most often and most comfortably. Do not be driven too far from this look. On the other hand, if you are not sufficiently defined, you will be so unfocused in your choices that nothing quite looks or feels like it was meant for you.

It's All in the Movement

An interesting way to form a visual perception of your look is to ask yourself, if you were a dance, what kind of dance would you be? Would you be jazz, flamenco, ballet, folk, waltz, fox trot, Charleston, twist, or something else? You do not need to be a dancer to picture each form of dance in your mind. What does each dance say about the dancer? How are the moves defined? Do you know someone who would fit into each category? Probably. Take time to feel the differences each dance form suggests to you.

For example, if you were to consider yourself a jazz dance and your best friend a ballet, you probably love more severe lines and colors while your friend loves more frilly, soft, feminine items. Take time to explore the possibilities. When you are in tune with your own music, you will find it easier to focus on the items that move with your personality. Could someone, given the list of dances, correctly guess which you represented? That is the goal!

Strike a Pose

Let your style suggest who you are. Do you have a look by which you are already known? Do not fight this look, emphasize it! For example, do you adore cats and own multiple clothing and accessory items that feature cats? Go ahead, take this passion a step further by collecting *even more* cat motifs. Become known as a cat lady. Possible versions of this "collectible" look are as limitless as your imagination. For example:

Be a "sweatshirt lady."
Be a "rose lady."
Be a "brooch lady."
Be an "eyeglass lady."
Be an "animal print lady."

Do you have a favorite color? For instance, maybe you wear a lot of blue. Make blue your signature color. Buy more blue on purpose. Become known as the "blue lady."

You can probably name someone that fits into a distinctive type. Contrary to what you may think, it is a compliment to your style for someone to pick an item off a rack and say, "Oh, this looks like you."

Do a personal inventory. Are you known for a particular passion? Do you raise orchids, ride horses, collect shells, fly kites, or love clowns? Do you garden, drive fast cars, volunteer at school, or have a passion for shoes? Both things you love and things you do can suggest a signature look. Take a moment to assess your pleasures and your collections.

I love to _____

_____

I collect _____

_____

Is there any way to translate this knowledge into your fashion presentation? The easiest form of expression is to dress to your current passions. Pick something you love, and use it over and over. People will talk to you and about you. Let what you love make you a standout.

Other tools can guide your way to finding your own special look. In the next section, we'll explore your fashion personality.

The Big Four

Fashion consultants have identified several clothing formulas that send signals about your basic lifestyle and personality. Filling out the following checklists will reveal how your personality shines through your dressing choices. Check *every* space that applies to you not just occasionally but often.

1

_____ You use conservative makeup.

_____ You wear conservative jewelry/accessories (pearls are your favorite).

_____ You have a controlled, "on purpose" hairdo.

_____ You prefer tailored clothing.

_____ You can't own too many basics.

_____ You wear paisley, dots, tone on tone patterns, plaid.

_____ You prefer soft materials such as silk, jersey, blends.

_____ You prefer understated style and consistency.

_____ You relate to Grace Kelly, Jackie Onassis, Princess Di, and Meryl Streep as role models.

2

_____ You wear little or no makeup.

_____ You wear little or no jewelry.

_____ You prefer a wash-and-wear hairstyle.

_____ You wear textured clothing.

_____ You prefer stripes, plaids, checks.

_____ You love denim.

_____ You love "masculine" clothing.

____ You shun fussy clothes.

____ You relate to Greta Garbo, Julia Roberts, and Katharine Hepburn as role models.

3

____ You love to experiment.

____ You love makeup.

____ You prefer angular haircuts.

____ You live in geometric and animal prints.

____ You wear contrasting colors.

____ Your jewelry is bold and exotic.

____ You aren't finished dressing until you have added some glitz.

____ You have a Type A personality.

____ You relate to Cher, Diana Ross, and Auntie Mame as role models.

4

____ You love makeup.

____ You wear your hair in a soft style.

____ You love subdued florals and pastels.

____ You prefer soft, flowing materials and ruffles.

____ You wear intricate jewelry.

____ You like to change your look.

____ You wear curved patterns such as flowers, bows, leaves, hearts, and butterflies.

____ You are dainty and feminine.

____ You favor Jane Seymour, Marilyn Monroe, and Dolly Parton as your role models.

Total the check marks within each category and write the numbers here:

1. _____ 2. _____ 3. _____ 4. _____

The category with the highest points is your basic look. The other categories, in descending order, are your accent groups. For instance, if you score highest in number 3, read more about your best look by going directly to Type 3. After reading your basic section, return to read about your accent types by turning to your second highest category, then your third and finally fourth categories.

Type 1: Traditional, Classic, Tailored

Whatever you call it—traditional, classic, or tailored—this category represents a majority of American women. If this is your style, the signature piece of clothing in your closet is the basic blazer. A traditional dresser could be considered a blazer collector. She has a closet full of tailored jackets, often several in the same color. If a blazer is your natural default dressing choice, you know you can't go wrong. Or can you?

As a second-fifty-year woman, gauge the continued appropriateness of your look by the reaction of the public. While holding fashion seminars, I have heard a familiar refrain: "I seem to have become invisible. Everybody seems to look right through me. It is like I have disappeared." Women seem to note this "disappearance" most commonly around sixty to sixty-five years of age.

If this problem rings true for you, whatever your age, it is time to reevaluate whether your look may now be too

The "Classic" look

conservative and safe. As nature creates a softer you, your clothing must become bolder to balance your presence. Remember, your goal is to be seen.

Buying ever more expensive blazers can enhance your look. There is something about money spent on clothing that shows. Don't be afraid to upgrade to more expensive blazers in your two or three favorite colors. An almost decadent dollar amount may be required, but this approach works wonders. The cut and fabric will be powerful, and as you know, a blazer is forever. Therefore, it's a great place to "invest" in you.

Another way to power up your current wardrobe is to borrow power from the other styles. You might wear bolder earrings or add ruffles. The unusual, the unexpected, adds sizzle, and sizzle is a great goal for a classic dresser. Fight looking boring. You must work to retain the power of youth. Explore becoming a refined eccentric.

Type 2: Natural, Sporty

You love casual, easy living and probably golf, bike, or garden for recreation. Your clothing suggests that you are athletic even though you may not be. You honor your practical side and may keep favorite items until they completely fall apart. I find in my seminars that sporty dressers often feel that they have no definable style. With a little extra attention to detail, sporty is its own distinctive style.

A true sporty woman must keep it simple. Fussing too much about clothes ruins the fun. On the

The "Sporty" look

138

other hand this is the style that can look neglectful so take particular care or you may look underdressed. Be sure that your hair, though carefree to manage, has a superb cut. Something as simple as using bolder earrings may be all that is needed. Natural stone necklaces add strength without being too "girly."

As a Sporty, every detail must count because you are *never* overdone. The best addition to this type is *attitude*. Wear it as an accessory!

Type 3: Exotic, Dramatic, Drama Queen, Diva

Everyone sees you coming because you can't imagine being a shy wallflower. You are independent and fiercely loyal. You are always "on stage" and just naturally make an entrance rather than simply enter a room. There is usually only one queen in any room—you. You plan it that way. You are always a head turner and have been known to accessorize even when working in the yard! You naturally gravitate toward any interesting look you don't already own, especially if you haven't seen it on anyone else. You almost live to dress. You are the enemy of understatement. If a Dramatic owns a blazer, it is beaded or sports an unusual cut. Your jewelry is oversized to match your personality and is often the star of your look. You love glitz and glamour. Bold color is your friend. What others may save for a special occasion, you wear daily.

Dramatics do not disappear at any age, but they may need to tone the look down

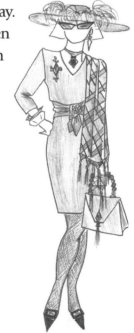

The "Dramatic" look

to a more sophisticated presentation over time. Then again, maybe not.

Dramatics are the women who give everyone else permission to be individuals because next to a Dramatic, you can never look overdone. Her yellow feather boa makes your new dangle earrings look almost traditional!

A Dramatic embraces being the "peppercorn in the stew of life." For her, less is never more, and more is never too much!

Type 4: Romantic, Feminine

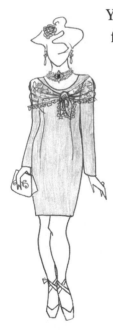

The "Romantic" look

You are the quintessential lady—soft, gentle, feminine. Your style evokes a sultry southern day. "Belle-ism" is a word you understand, even if it is not in the dictionary. Your strength is in your superfemininity. You rule through your smile. You think ruffles were invented just for you, and you love the sensual feeling of flowing materials against your body. Your closet is full of soft lines and breezy fabrics.

You are never overdone, and your colors are soft. Your style is the perfect accent to all the other styles. Especially as women age, a more feminine mystique is becoming. A beauty in her eighties and nineties naturally stands out in her gentle, always detailed, Romantic look.

Note how slight differences in detail can create a new style:

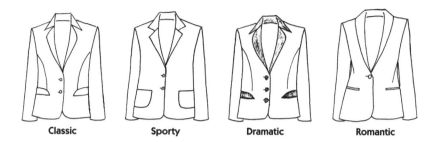

| Classic | Sporty | Dramatic | Romantic |

Combining Styles

Most women wear a combination of styles with one dominant. The danger, if you are equally involved with each type, is that you have not focused on a style of your own and instead may be buying everything you see. Discern your style. Invest in it. Accessorize from the other styles. For instance, Dolly Parton could be seen as a Natural/Sporty because she has an earthy cowgirl flair and looks so good in denim. She is also a Romantic/Feminine because she adds lace and ruffles and has lots of hair. Her hyperfemininity determines that her true type is Romantic/Feminine, but she accents with Natural/Sporty fabrics.

You will know you have found your style when *you* wear your clothing, it doesn't wear you. Each style works for someone. Be sure yours works for you. If this exercise has entertained and edified you, good. If it has only confused and overwhelmed you, that is natural too. It may be worth your time and money to hire a personal shopper or image coach for a few hours to help you pull your best look together. Image coaches do this for a living because they love their work but also because so many people need their help.

There is no shame in needing a little one-on-one time with a consultant. After working with this book, you will have a better idea how to use these services. If you are considering hiring a personal shopper or image coach, you'll find more information in the appendix.

Step into Style, Then Step Out

Here's a great checklist from *Branding Yourself* by Mary Spillane, also the author of *Color Me Beautiful*. Stand in front of a full-length mirror and look yourself over before you go out. Answer yes or no to each of these statements. Remember, your look includes all your physical features, your grooming style, and your clothing choices.[1]

_____ Your look is just that, yours.
_____ Your friends expect to see you like this.
_____ At best, you are more. Your choices enhance your best bits.
_____ You are at ease and look it.
_____ Your grooming is complete and appears effortless.
_____ Nothing jars. Your look is in balance.
_____ Nothing is contrived.
_____ You have "fine" touches.
_____ You look like you took care in dressing.
_____ You do not fuss with your clothes, no tugging or pulling.
_____ Your look is now but timeless.

If you've carried out your look well, people want to know you *because of how you look* even before you open your mouth. Practice using this checklist until putting your look together is a habit.

This checklist is also a great exercise to play with your friends. Getting feedback about your best looks is powerfully affirming. Point by point, ask each other, "What does this statement mean?" Then, "How does one make that point more strongly?" Learn from and with your friends. When you see how differences in taste make for a more interesting world, you will have more confidence in your own contribution.

All about "It"

The ability to project a strong image is sometimes referred to as having "it." When you have *it*, you have power. You stand uniquely alone in a crowd even when the crowd is full of others who have *it*. When you have *it*, you have presence. Who in your circle has *it*? *It* comes with being *seen*. Make *it* yours.

Chapter 11

Flattering Style:
Tricks for the Second Fifty Years

*B*efore addressing your specific figure type in the next chapter, you need to be aware of figure changes that affect nearly everyone eventually and simple visual tricks you can use to minimize the shift.

Your time to experience these physical changes may still be on the horizon or these issues may affect you directly today. There is even a chance these issues will never touch you, but a general awareness is educational.

You have heard of "ideal" proportions and you lived your first fifty years aware of how closely you fit those ideals. Welcome to a time when *everybody* is shifting away from the ideal. You'll probably find little comfort in the fact that the masses are here with you. That's why this is another of those "just get over it" lessons.

Understanding why something happens—such as changes in body proportions—can make it more acceptable. The big culprit? Earth's gravitational pull—as one ages, one gets closer to the ground. The longer you live, the more this pull draws you toward the earth's center. Because of gravity, you shorten as you get older. It is the natural result of a lifetime of fighting gravity to sit and walk upright. If you lived on the moon, your backbone would actually relax and expand as you got older rather than constrict.

On Earth, over time, your backbone shortens. So does your neck. So do your legs. Gravity is constant, and everyone's bones and joints eventually succumb to that pressure. What is individual is the degree of that shortening. Although members of the same family do not respond identically, genetics play a big role. (This is where years of exercise can pay great dividends.)

If bones respond to gravity like this, how much more do the soft tissues? Your body parts just don't sit or hang where they used to! Don't despair.

Mirror, Mirror on the Wall

That's enough of the facts about your figure changes. Let's move on to the tricks. First, using a full-length mirror is a must. Refusing to view your whole look can be disastrous. Use this mirror in your fight against gravity.

The Magic Lift

The number one exercise all second-fifty-year women need to do is this: stand in front of your full-length mirror, hook your thumbs under your bra straps, and *lift*. You just lost ten to fifteen years, didn't you? If you laughed to yourself, you ought to see what I

Use a full-length mirror!

146

see when I ask an audience to do this exercise. It
is as if the whole room gets a body lift.

Perform this procedure and adjust your
straps at least weekly. It is amazing how
straps give. Keep them high!

We may laugh, but this problem is serious. Create a mantra: I must adjust my bust. I
must adjust my bust.

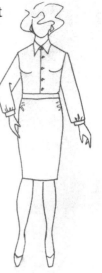

Neck and Neck

Your neck comes into play in two ways. Yes,
your neck shortens with age, like so many
other body parts. But of more immediate

The bust lift

concern is that your neck skin is the first to lose its elasticity.
Some women, in an effort to conceal this first sign of aging,
start to wear higher-necked tops or to button their blouses to
the top. This trick works for a few short years,
then it becomes counterproductive.

Open your blouse and look. Your last,
very best, most unwrinkled skin is on your
chest. It never had much fat under it; it
never stretched, so it never wrinkles. If you
have not had serious sun damage to the area
and if you have no significant surgical scar-
ring, then this is an area to be shown off. It
is the perfect background for a beautiful
piece of jewelry. In short, open-collared
blouses are an elongating, youthful look.
Second-fifty-year women everywhere,

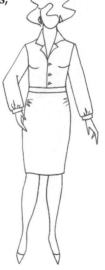

The open collar

undo those buttons and show a little skin!

When adding shells and T-shirts to your wardrobe, consider the V neck, but a few other interesting necklines also create wonderful lines. These necklines come under the heading of "guilt-free shopping" because they are not always easy to find. When you do, grab them!

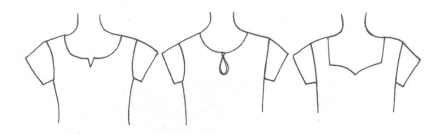

Show a little skin!

Put Your Shoulders into It

Your shoulders are especially prone to showing the effects of gravity. Straight, solid shoulders are a mark of youth. They represent power and vitality. They also assure that your clothing drapes properly. What does gravity do? It tends, over time, to pull your wonderful shoulders earthward.

At this age, shoulder pads are your friend—not as a fashion statement but as a way to fill in the space gravity has created between you and a solid shoulder line. A *few* women never need them. Lucky them. The rest of us *must* use them. Shoulder pads "lift" your body silhouette back to a more youthful look. You should own several sizes and colors of shoulder pads and add them to any top that comes without them.

If you are unsure as to your need for these fashion friends, it can be helpful to look at photos of yourself in your twenties.

Now, step once again in front of your full-length mirror. Insert a shoulder pad on only one side. Which side looks more like your youthful self? Find a pad size that helps you regain your former shoulder line. Your clothes will fit better and people will notice the difference, although they will not know what has changed.

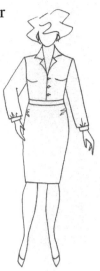

If you have tops with shoulder pads attached with Velcro, remove them from the intended top and use them in your "padless" tops. For most tops, you will not need the opposing Velcro strip to stabilize the pad. The strip on the pad will grip the shoulder

Shoulder pads

seam of the garment. Experiment. You don't want wandering pads to trail behind you at some event.

Waist Not

Moving down the body to your waist, keep in mind that tucking in your top is one of the biggest mistakes you can make if your waist has shortened. Look in your mirror. If your shoulders are rounding, your waist is shortening. If you are losing height, your waist is shortening. As soon as you tuck and belt yourself around the middle, you have created a visual "stop" in a place that is not your intended focus. It may have been a great look for you at twenty years of age, but not now.

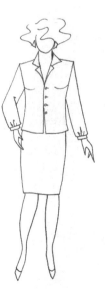

Relaxed waist

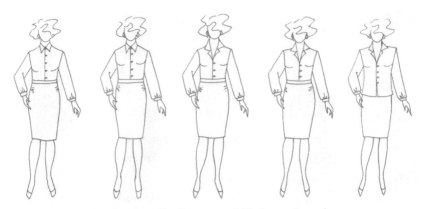

A series of small adjustments yields dramatic results

Gaining weight at any age also serves to shorten the waist. Look honestly at yourself in your full-length mirror again. Are you in proportion? The most flattering look divides your body into thirds from top to bottom. If your top is less than one-third of your total body silhouette when you tuck in a shirt, it is time to stop tucking. If you wish to wear a belt, use a belt designed to fall over the hip and/or belt it over an un-tucked top. An implied waist can be much more attractive.

Create a "virtual" waist with pushed-up sleeves. Look in a mirror. With your long sleeves down, your shape is what it is. Now push your sleeves up near your elbows, and you have vi-sually created an hourglass figure. The eye sees broad shoul-ders (including your upper arms) then passes to lower arm level to your small "waist." The eye follows the line of your clothing, finishing at your wider hips. Easy and effective!

Looking Good

A flattering fit is just that, flattering. Is there anything more miserable than wearing something that is too tight? Clothing that is "stressed" at some point creates a visual stop right at the

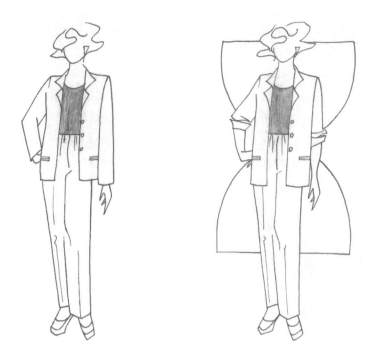

point you probably wish would be ignored. Be very careful that the fit of your clothing is friendly and relaxed. When your clothing feels friendly, you feel friendly, and suddenly, everyone around you seems friendly. Don't let your clothing make you miserable—because it can.

Be Hip

You want your impression to focus on your positive aspects. There are a few tricks in this department too. If you carry your weight through the hips, never button your jacket or sweater across your fullest point. Unbuttoning relaxes your look. Also be careful that your open tops do not pull back at the bottom, as this again will misdirect the focus downward toward the wrong stop. If you wear a matching pant and top under your open jacket or sweater, you gain visual height as the eye is drawn up, uninterrupted, to your face.

With this trick, you have also inadvertently practiced the "Rule of Three." This rule suggests that adding a third piece to your top-bottom combination is slimming. The third piece allows your figure to be suggested rather than defined. The eye flows upward and the emphasis ends where you want it to, at

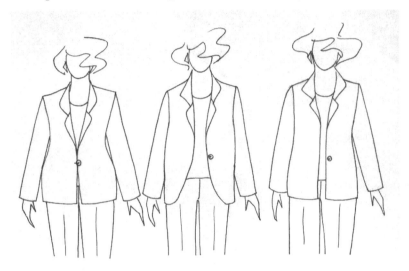

your smile. Your third piece could be a blouse, jacket, vest, or necklace. The third piece creates balance.

Remember this fact: the eye sweeps then stops at the point of heaviest emphasis. Add weight to your outfit so that you bring the eye to your best bits and away from your challenges. This idea is addressed in depth in the next chapter.

Simple Dressing

Simplicity is foolproof. Start your day dressed in a basic pant and matching shell. Wearing all one color, so the eye is not stopped, is very lengthening and flattering. Now stand in front of your closet and pick any jacket, blouse, sweater, or scarf that suits your fancy. You can't go wrong. The matching top and bottom elongate your look while the Rule of Three also comes into play. Watch how many stylish women you see on television and in the mall that have used this simple trick.

Tapered slacks provide a taller illusion than a wide leg. Hips also appear smaller with this silhouette. Wear your waistbands loose enough so that they sit just below your natural waistline. If the waistband is too tight, it will create a balloon effect right where you do not want to focus attention. Waistbands should fit so that you can comfortably slip two fingers between you and the band. You will always be safe if you refer to the "Two Pieces of Pie Rule." It states: if you can eat two pieces of pie at Thanksgiving and not want to cut your waistband through in six places, you probably have the right fit!

Your style is right when it shows your best assets and makes them the stars. Knowing that those around you see you in the very best light is your reward. Be confident. Your confidence will be contagious, and the world will thank you.

Don't be shy. When you are experimenting with your style, don't be afraid it is "too much." As Mae West said, "It is better to get looked over than to get overlooked."[1] You'll never learn if you don't allow yourself to make a few mistakes. You are only playing dress-up, after all.

You have one more assignment in front of your full-length mirror: blow yourself a kiss!

Chapter 12

Proper Fit: Keeping It Friendly

*Y*ou need to define yourself as a *physical* size and body type. With this knowledge comes power—the power of knowing your most flattering silhouettes, hence the power to be seen.

Showing Your Stuff

Is your weight in flux? Do you have several different sizes in your closet? Do you buy your wished-for size or your actual size? As of today, when you shop, promise yourself one thing: "I will buy for the size and weight I am *now*."

If you are not on a diet program but think you will lose weight so that a smaller size will fit, get over it. Buy for today. If you are on a diet program, nothing looks worse than something purchased too small and worn too soon. If you are losing weight, you need clothes for the transition. Buy for where you are now.

Whether you are planning to lose weight or are happy "as is," remember that you look slimmer if your clothes fit easily. The more they hug you, the larger you appear. Keep your fit friendly. Friendly clothes hug your assets and flow over your challenges. When you try on a garment, stand, sit, turn, and reach. A friendly fit allows your clothing to flow with your movement rather than tug against your movement. Unimpeded movement lets the eye rest on your best bits and ignore the challenges.

Size is not the only determinant of a proper fit. Your specific body type must also be addressed.

Body Type

You probably have something about your figure that you would love to change, but that change won't happen today and maybe it never will. It may be little consolation, but you are not alone with your particular issues. What is a girl to do? How do you make your style look put together, not thrown together? The short answer is to dress *into* your challenges or dress *around* your challenges.

You may have seen charts of triangles, rectangles, and so on used to define body types. These shapes work as illustrations, but they are no fun. Your inner girl wants to have fun and demands her value be acknowledged. She loves herself unconditionally and knows she is of rare value. Her body is a natural part of this package. What item in nature can best represent her treasure? Diamonds!

It is said that a diamond is a girl's best friend, and you should be your own best friend by now. That logically makes you a diamond. The clearer the diamond, the higher its value. It is the same with humans. The better you know yourself, the more you have to give and the greater your positive impact. It is of no small consequence that the larger the diamond, the greater its value.

In the diamond industry, any diamond other than round is referred to as "fancy shaped." There is usually a premium paid for these shapes. You too have a fancy shape that is part of your own unique, fancy package. Be fancy, think fancy, have a fancy attitude. Do you feel it?

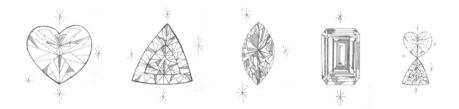

Accept yourself where you are today. What fancy shape are you? To assure proper fit and body-type analysis, you must first understand "stops" and determine your "critical measurement."

Stops

It is natural for the human eye to follow motion. We observe people without being fully aware that we are constantly scanning our surroundings. As part of this scan-and-be-scanned universe, you need to be aware of something called "stops." Stops occur at the point of greatest presence, whether in diamonds, architecture, nature, or the human figure. Look at the diamond shapes above. Notice how your eyes first scan the shape, then return and settle on the "heaviest" point of the diamond. Likewise, we observers are first caught by some unique detail, be it size, color, or sparkle. Unconsciously, we do a foot-to-head scan and then settle back on the "heaviest" point or out-of-balance center and stop. Notice how the emerald cut leads you to perform multiple scans as there is no stop to this shape. Where our figures are concerned, our critical measurement determines our natural stop.

Critical Measurement

Good news! You can dress to balance away from your physical stop whenever you wish, but first you must find your critical measurement. Use this simple test: when you put on a box-cut jacket, where does the fit *fail* you?

If the jacket pulls through the bust, you are a heart fancy shape and your bustline is your stop. If the jacket pulls through the middle, then you are a marquise fancy shape and your waist is your stop. If the jacket pulls through the hip, you are a trilliant fancy shape and your hipline is your stop. If the jacket fits equally well at all points but you do not have a small waist, you are an emerald-cut fancy shape and your issue becomes not having a stop. To you hourglass girls, who have a small waist, you will get recognition later in this chapter, so keep reading.

Getting Fancy

Fancy is as fancy does. There are several wonderful ways for diamonds to be cut. All are beautiful and treasured. Add the diamond to your list of totems for it clearly represents a small portion of your true value, importance, and rarity. The ability to become more brilliant is in your hands. Start by finding your fancy shape.

The Heart

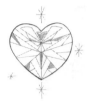

Your critical measurement is your bust. This shape is not a boring inverted triangle but a loving work of art. It has a natural sophisticated aura. Strong shoulders, so desirable, are a natural to this body type. Very small hips mean that much detail can be focused in this area to good effect. If you are a heart-cut fancy shape, good for you!

Your greatest challenge: minimizing the bustline stop.

The Trilliant

Your critical measurement is your hip. This body shape is not a pear, not a who-cares triangle, but a trilliant-cut fancy shape! It's much more festive, desirable, and brilliant. A trilliant is narrow at the top and dramatically expands toward the bottom. This is a very beautiful shape for cut diamonds and a natural shape for human females. This is the shape that best suits childbirth and the replenishment of the earth. Ample hips are a good feature. If you are a trilliant-cut fancy shape, good for you!

Your greatest challenge: balancing the shoulders to reduce the hip stop.

The Marquise

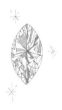

Your critical measurement is your waist. This body shape is not an apple, not a meaningless circle, but a marquise-cut fancy shape! This body type has a comfortable, warm, cuddly aspect. Honor this fancy shape and she has so much to give. Her lap is often holding the wounded children of the world. If you are a marquise-cut fancy shape, good for you!

Your greatest challenge: finding slacks with a low front rise.

The Emerald Cut

 The critical measurement test is easy for you to pass. This body type is not a rectangle but an emerald cut. This is an easy figure to dress. An emerald-cut figure is balanced at every weight. Lucky her, this type gains and loses equally on the top and bottom. The fact that her waist is not as defined as the hourglass is okay because she is a diamond, after all. Why would she want to whittle away something so valuable? If you are an emerald-cut fancy shape, good for you!

Your greatest challenge: creating a waist stop.

The Hourglass

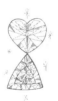 This body type is always the "ideal" yet it makes up such a small percentage of the natural female form. It seems all fashion was designed with this body type in mind. She has the shoulders of the heart cut and the hips of the trilliant cut, but her waist is all her own. If you are an hourglass, good for you! Naturally, it takes two diamond cuts to represent you.

Your greatest challenge: staying humble.

If you have found your symbol, you are ready to maximize your strengths by creating multiple stops to balance your challenges. Turn to the section that addresses your own fancy shape. (Sorry, hourglasses, there's no section for you since you can wear virtually anything that fits. There is no right or wrong look.) This chapter is meant to guide you to a basic understanding of your best looks. Do not bother with other shapes at this point, as the goal is to develop a clear image of your own personal look and the two or three tricks necessary to maximize your assets.

Here's to You If You Are a Heart-Cut Fancy Shape!

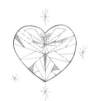 Those who have never had your critical measurement issue just don't understand the dilemma. A large bust is feminine, but a large bust is heavy to carry and is too often the center of attention. Those with naturally small breasts have no idea of the difficulty you have getting and maintaining eye contact. An oversized bust can be like an attention-grabbing sibling that you wish would let you have center stage more often.

To dress *into* a large bust is to leave the attention on the bust and be overtly sexy. That is always a choice. To dress *around* a large bust is to balance attention over the whole person. Some days you will choose one and some the other. Either way you must start with a properly fitted bra. Spend your first fashion dollars here.

Bless you if you have broad shoulders. You may have rued their strength in days past, but they are one of your greatest assets today. Love them and dress into them. On the other hand, if you have narrow shoulders with an ample bust, you must add shoulder pads to balance your figure. Under no circumstance are you to cut pads out of your blouses or jackets. (This is one exception to the "rules are only suggestions" mantra we espouse. This rule *rules*.) The power to manage a large bust begins with a strong shoulder line.

If your bustline has received more than its due share of attention, it is time to divert the attention to other areas of the body. Start by increasing the use of accessories at the neckline. Open your neckline to reveal more skin above the bust. Showcase heavy pieces of jewelry against this skin. Increase the size of your earrings and let your hair, if possible, provide substantial heft.

Next, you are free to increase the interest around your hip area. You absolutely shine in broomstick skirts and wear pleated skirts in heavy fabrics very effectively.

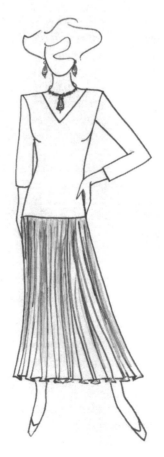

You are also the one who can most successfully wear bright-print fabrics in your bottom pieces. Overblouses and jackets should be long enough to cover the hip and taper in at the bottom. Otherwise, there is a danger that you will appear pregnant. Since most tops are cut straight up and down, you can use a decorative pin at the hip to add a downward-focused stop as well as a better fit.

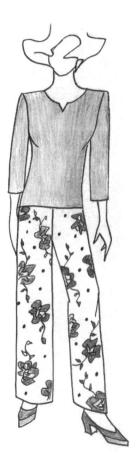

Embroidery detail at the hip is also very balancing, as is three-piece dressing. When you add a jacket, your bust has to play peek-a-boo to be noticed. All of the detail in this outfit leads the eye back to you. If you love interesting shoes, make them part of your signature. In this illustration, the bustline is the weakest of multiple stops from shoes to ankle treatment to hip treatment to neck treatment.

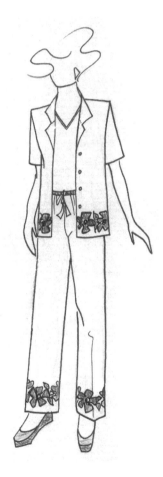

For more traditional dressing, the third piece, here a vest, elongates your look by guiding the eye up the center of your figure. The eye sees the opening as your figure. It is important that this third piece does not pull but comfortably lies across your bustline to create a straight up-and-down scan.

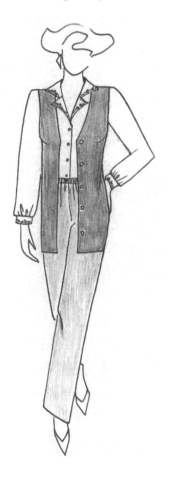

Adding interest to the neck detail finishes the stop at the face. For those who eschew jewelry, purchasing tops with embroidered collars produces the same effect. These embroidered basics can be considered "preaccessorized" and take some of the terror out of putting a whole look together.

In the final analysis, dear heart-cut fancy shape, love your shoulders, love your bust, love your hips, love your legs because you perfectly reflect your whole being and it is fabulous!

You're a Trilliant-Cut Fancy Shape and You're Fabulous!

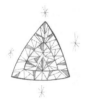

You are shaped to birth babies whether you ever do or not. You see fashion items on models that you love and somehow the item fails miserably on you. Welcome to *my* world! Luckily, a good strong hipline has, in recent years, become far more fashionable.

As a trilliant-cut fancy shape you can choose to dress *into* a well-shaped derriére or *around* a less-than-perfect stop. Do not be afraid to list your bottom as one of your favorite bits. At the very least, a strong hipline usually means that you can sit comfortably for longer periods of time than your hip-challenged sisters.

Still, all in all, balance is desired. The operative word here is *shoulders*. To a trilliant-cut fancy shape, shoulder pads are absolutely essential, not as a fashion statement but as figure-balancing friends. Collect a wardrobe of shoulder pads in multiple sizes in natural, black, and white. Shoulder pads aid in bringing the final stop back to your face.

With proper shoulder pads, the blazer or box jacket flatters your proportions. First, never button your jacket across your critical measurement. If you do, you create a tummy stop that is hard to balance. Leave your jackets open. The scanning eye moves freely up toward the face without a hip stop. Second, bring your naturally small waist back visually by wearing your sleeves pushed up. Finally, contrasting colored or print tops further ask the scanning eye to pause on your smaller upper half.

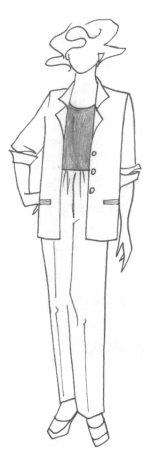

The big shirt is designed to echo the length of the blazer without being so formal. Make sure this shirt comfortably covers your hips, then add shoulder pads to balance your silhouette. Determine your favorite colors, then purchase matching slacks and shells as your basic "under group." When you start the morning with a unicolored, two-piece set, you can safely stand in front of your closet, half-asleep, select any shirt or jacket, and know you have created an outfit that works. Adding jewelry and neck treatments add visual weight that makes the final stop at or near your face.

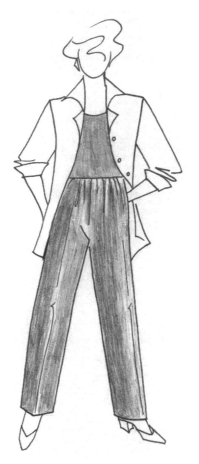

A short jacket with a dynamic hourglass cut works very well for some trilliant figures. Make sure that the shoulders of the jacket are especially strong and the waist is nipped in. The one button leads the eye to the waist, a good stop for the trilliant as long as the whole silhouette balances the hip line. You might ask a friend if you look as good walking away as you do approaching!

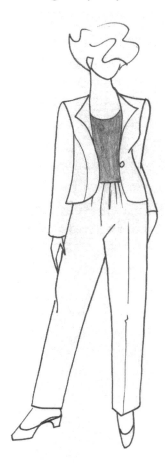

Three-piece dressing, whether with slacks or skirts, is always friendly to the trilliant-cut fancy shape. If you choose skirts, they generally need to hug your hip until they fall below your fullest point. A gored skirt is a very soft beautiful balance for the trilliant hipline. When you wear a belt, let it rest on your hip rather than cinch around your waist. A too-small waist in proportion to your hips will be distracting. With a tie belt, as pictured, wear the tie to one side, not down the middle. The off-center position of the belt shortens the scan from left to right and creates a narrower hip stop.

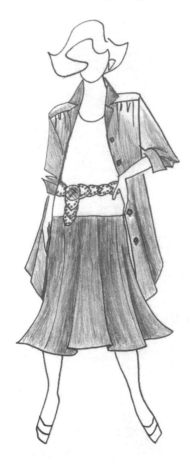

Feel free to create stops at your feet with interesting shoes, at your legs with fancy hose, at your bust with ruffles and color, and of course at your neck and face with accessories. If you are uncomfortable with accessories, fill your wardrobe with tops that have wonderful embroidery at the neck or shoulder level. This detail creates a natural stop without further input from you. Patterned bottoms and fancy hip treatments are not completely off limits but do take a trained eye to assure the balance of your silhouette has not been disturbed.

Well, beautiful trilliant-cut fancy shape, love yourself as a wonderful, feminine female form. Create fabulous stops right where you want them because you deserve to be seen!

You're a Marquise-Cut Fancy Shape—
These Pages Are for You!

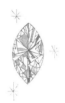 How unfair! Big breasts and big hips can be construed as desirable but never a large waist. This issue is another one of those "just get over it" issues. After all, the marquise-cut diamond far outsells the heart-cut and trilliant-cut fancy shapes. You are a diamond now, girlfriend, and within the human species your shape is normal and customary. From today forward, step out with a diamond attitude for your figure represents a desired form.

Since the waist is a stop you wish to minimize, try some natural silhouettes that do exactly that. The number one friendly cut for your figure is the banded jacket often referred to as a "baseball" jacket. This jacket look creates a soft added dimension that allows extra fabric to cover the waist while creating a stop at your smaller hip line. How perfect! Wear shells and bottoms in matching colors. You will create an elongating up-and-down scan with your waist taken out of the equation. Be very careful about tucking in your shells. It works for some but not other marquises.

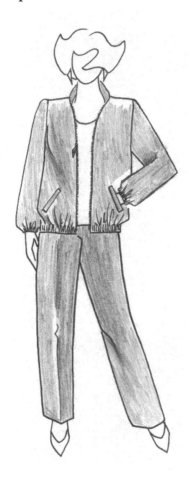

Tunic blouses work very well also, especially the artist's smock style. The extra fabric in this style allows for a comfortable motion over and around your figure. Wear unicolor shell-and-pant sets under your tops to keep the scanning eye moving toward your face. Adding bold jewelry and shoulder treatments will create a final stop.

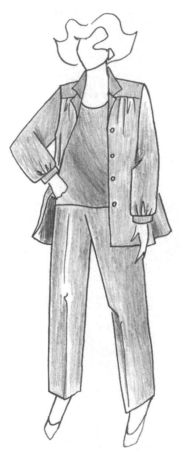

Be very careful with T-shirts. If they are just pulled down straight, your waist will take center stage. If you tease the eye with an offsetting diagonal line, your waist returns to its proper balance. This look works equally well with slacks and skirts. If you are wearing a skirt, see that it tapers in at the bottom to create balance. Full skirts can be overpowering and should be avoided unless you have a trained eye.

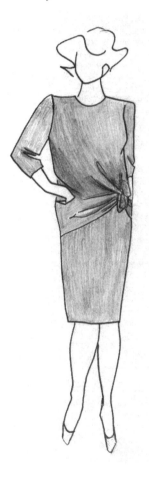

Casual, loose-fitting dresses are your friends. Let them be bold and fun because you are bold and fun. Enjoy the freedom of movement. Team little sundresses with a three-quarter-sleeve tee for a very current, young look. Add sassy earrings and you are ready to go!

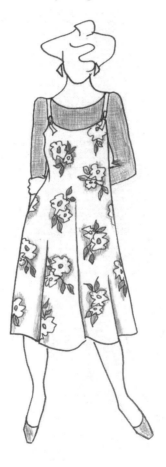

Have fun creating stops at your feet with great shoes, at your calves with capris, at your neck and shoulders with embroidered delights or funky jewelry. Wear big glasses and great hats. Develop a really big attitude toward life. You, my dear, have fabulous gifts to give and have every right, and yes, responsibility, to say, "Hey! Look at me!"

Here's to You, Emerald-Cut Fancy Shape!

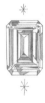 You are a great shape to dress and you should give yourself credit for having a great, desirable figure. The beauty of the emerald-cut fancy shape is that heavier or thinner, your hips and shoulders are always in proportion. You never have to rebalance yourself; you just buy clothes that fit!

If you lack anything worth noting, it would be your waistline, an easy visual fix. You many not have the waist of the hourglass type, but you have everything else. It is easy to fake a waistline so nobody knows the difference. Lucky you!

When you want a waist, create that stop on your outfit. Here, simply tying your shirttails creates a heavy stop right where you want your physical impression magnified. Wearing a shell under your blouse and leaving the blouse open creates a V point so the eye scans to the waist then back to the face where you want your final stop.

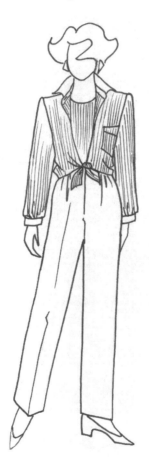

Because of the great balance to your figure, you can wear two-piece outfits with abandon. There is no need for a waist with this look, but if you want to create the illusion for your own satisfaction, add a dynamic belt just below your natural waistline. Your belts should rest gently on your hip with any tie placed off center. The off-center tie causes the eye to make a narrow scan left to right, causing a slimmer effect.

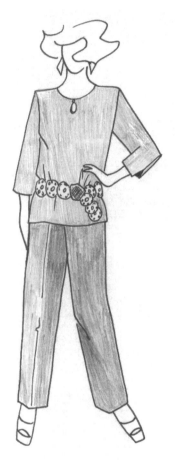

Wear tailored jackets that don't nip too tightly through the waist. The lines on this jacket suggest a small waist, although it is a straight cut. Add a small belt over the jacket to create a visual definition of your waist.

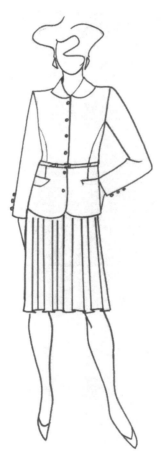

Everything about this outfit points to a wonderfully small waist. The shirt is tucked in; the vest is open and tailored with darts. Because the vest drops lightly over your actual waistline, no one knows that there isn't an hourglass figure under there! This is the Rule of Three in action, and it works wonderfully for you. The vest, as the third piece, hides what you don't want seen while suggesting the waist you do want seen.

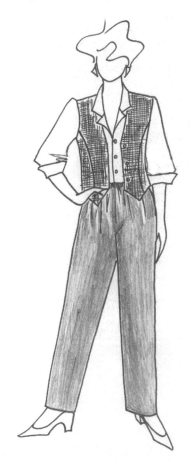

Lucky you, your body is your playground! You get to create stops wherever you please. Feel free to spotlight your feet, calves, legs, hips, or bust at will. You can wear trim and embellishment wherever you wish.

When you have finished costuming, step back to scan your whole look. In the end, it is your face we want as a final stop. Your outfit should be interesting wherever the eye journeys, but leave the greatest emphasis to stop at your sparkling eyes and beautiful smile!

The Final Details

Proper fit certainly includes proper pant length. Unless your slacks were designed to be "cropped," be sure they are long enough. Here are the rules, and they do apply, especially for second-fifty-year women.

- Tapered: This most flattering, lengthening cut is worn a little shorter than a straight cut. Because of the taper, the hem should just barely drop over the back of your shoe and touch your instep. Having a small "break" or fold at the instep is also acceptable.
- Straight cut: This look should reach halfway down the back of your shoe and gently rest on the top of your foot at the front.
- Palazzo or full cut: This pant should cover the back of your shoe to the point where the upper meets the heel. It will be correspondingly longer in front also. These pants are often worn as evening slacks.

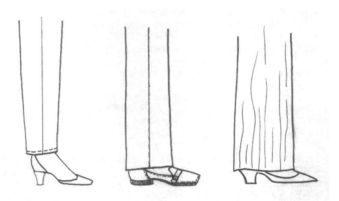

Shine On

You, diamond girl, now have a clarity of vision and under-standing of cut to find the best silhouettes to maximize your presence. You are having more fun playing dress-up because you know the tricks that make it easy. Hug your wonderful fancy shape and know that what you have and who you are is more than enough. Diamonds are forever.

Chapter 13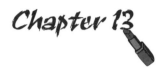

Eye Candy: Accessorizing to Amaze

*T*he *New World Dictionary* defines accessories as "something extra, a thing added to help in a secondary way."[1] This is true, sometimes. At other times, your accessories say more about you than your clothing.

What is your comfort zone for accessories? Does it change from day to day? Do you shun accessories because they are just too confusing? Then keep it simple with a few techniques that never fail. Pick a few pieces that can go with nearly every outfit. Accessorize to be seen.

About Your Face

All attention, in the end, should finish at your eyes and your smile. You can create this effect in numerous ways. Evaluate your accessory choices for their shine, motion, size, and shape.

Motion and Light

It is true that eyes follow motion and light. Since your goal is to be present and be seen, using accessories nearest your face is your first priority. Earrings are the natural guide between an observer and you. The second-fifty-year woman is well served by wearing earrings that dangle, even slightly, and/or catch the light in a way that attracts the eye. The earring itself does not need to be remarkable to garner the desired effect. Necklaces that complement these effects also promote an upward stop. Next time you are in a group, notice how many times your eyes are drawn toward just these features.

Make each purchase count. Look for basic colors or metals that will catch the light and provide motion. As you begin to accessorize, start with accent jewelry rather than venturing into "artwork" pieces. Those can be added to your wardrobe as you gain confidence in your ability to present yourself. It's okay to shock your friends, but you have gone too far when *you* are in shock over your choices! Accessorize to shock your friends when larger, artier pieces give you confidence, not trepidation.

Size

Second, consider size. Pick jewelry that fits within or just slightly outside *your* comfort zone. Remember, you want to feel confident, not foolish. In general, a bolder physical presence requires bolder accessories, and a more petite body shows well with smaller pieces. Still, if you are petite, own a few larger pieces, and if you are taller, occasionally wear smaller pieces. Be bold for you. Your inner girl loves accessorizing. Trust her.

Shape

Next, consider accessory shape. Look at any jewelry display and you will see many choices from soft and curved to

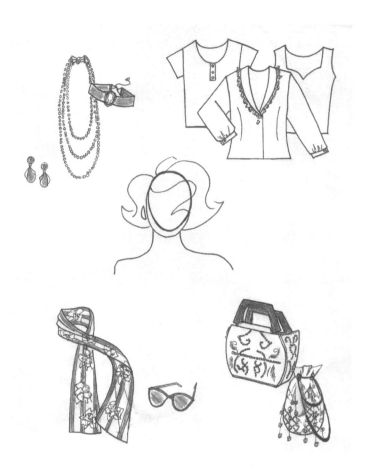

severely angular. What is your best choice in shape? Look no further than your own mirror for the answer. Is your face a softly curved round or oval? Or is your face a more angular square or rectangle?

When picking accessories, start by choosing those that echo your face shape. If your face is angular, pick angular earrings, necklaces, and scarf prints. If it's rounded, pick soft, curved pieces. Look at your current accessories. How many of your very favorite pieces are a repeat of your own lines?

Warning: do not throw out items that seem to conflict with this "rule." Sometimes the color of an accessory is of more

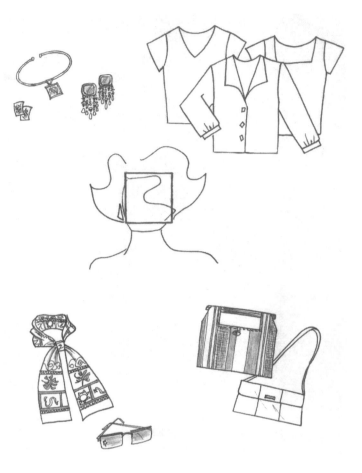

importance than the shape. At other times, the shape echoes a pattern in an outfit, therefore adding an extra dimension. With accessories in particular, the rules are only suggestions.

But, in general, consider your face shape when shopping for new accessories. If you can choose between several shapes in the color you need, honor your own natural lines and you cannot fail.

Take this concept one step further and echo these shapes in your clothing choices. Square necklines and angular collars may honor your natural lines, or choose soft curves. Look at the illustrations; now look at your wardrobe. You probably have some of these examples in your closet. Which are your favorites? Again, this is not a rule, only a direction you may favor when given both choices.

Accessory Wardrobes

Your clothing wardrobe is a collection of all the items you need to dress for the way you live. Have you planned your accessory wardrobes as carefully as your clothing wardrobe, or are there gaping holes in your collection?

On the simplest level, three basic accessory wardrobes can stylishly cover your needs. First is an accessory wardrobe that *matches* your hair, whether it's blonde, brunette, auburn, white, or salt-and-pepper. Collect earrings, necklaces, chokers, and scarves that are your exact hair color.

The second accessory wardrobe should be your metallic color. Again, look to your hair color for focus. If your hair is silver or salt-and-pepper, wear silver, especially around your face. If your hair is blonde or auburn, wear gold. A brunette with auburn streaks can wear either. Again, build a wardrobe of both real and faux pieces that bring you into focus. Do not be afraid to mix gold and silver when that look works with your outfit. Being overly matched is passé!

Your third basic accessory wardrobe should include the coloration of the "bottoms" you wear most frequently. If you wear navy pants or skirts, have a navy accessory wardrobe. The same is true for black, red, khaki, rose, or blue, whatever your favorite is. Adding your "bottom" color back near your face creates balance and a stop for the eye to settle on in its sweep of the interesting picture you present.

Spend a day going from store to store just trying on costume jewelry. Try both gentle and bold looks. Picture what outfits you might wear the pieces with. This isn't a time to buy unless you find some long sought-after piece. Look in magazines and even newspaper clothing circulars for current fashion looks. Bring out pieces you already own that make a statement.

Costume jewelry is fun and affordable, but it's not for everyone. If you wear minimal jewelry, it must be of the highest quality you can afford. Save and buy better pieces as you get older. If you are a minimalist Natural/Sporty type, you will find comfort in wearing natural stone pieces for a bolder look.

Neckwear

Necklaces and scarves also lead the eye to the wearer. Longer necklaces and long scarves will create an illusion of an elongated neck while shorter ones serve to "frame" the face.

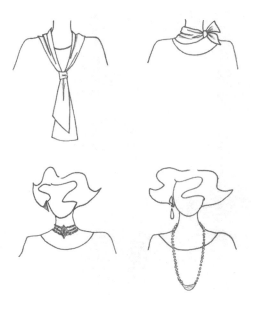

Own a few fabulous scarves. Whether you have a few or a lot, scarves are inexpensive add-ons that speak volumes about your look. Two very simple scarf ties will suffice to finish your look.

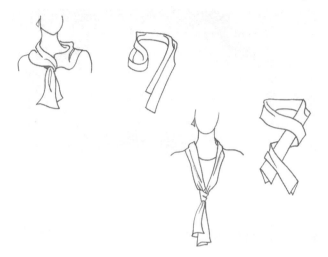

While we're discussing the neck, there are several T-shirt necklines that work as accessories in their own right. Add them to your wardrobe as you find them in your favorite colors.

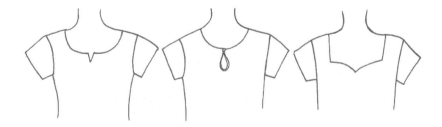

Guilt-Free Shopping

Accessories are the best vacation purchase. You can shop and shop without buying too much and when you find the perfect look, the items don't take up a lot of room in your luggage.

You can probably wear them with basic clothes you already have in your suitcase, and as a bonus, when you get home they make a fabulous memento from your trip. How great, when someone says, "I love your necklace," for you to be able to say, "Thank you! I found this while I was in New Orleans." You remember a good time and you have multiple conversational paths to follow from there. Accessories, properly collected, are great friends in any crowd.

Another way to get hours of fun shopping without spending much money is to look for the perfect accessory for one specific, unusual outfit already in your closet. You may be looking for a particular color or you may want a bolder impact. Do not compromise. Items that make up a perfect outfit can come together years apart. Buy what charms you.

Artistic Expression

When you accessorize, you are an artist. You may not be able to paint a masterpiece, but you can develop your eye to pick what makes *you* a masterpiece. Keep adding elements to your look until you have come into full focus. You may be retired, but forget about being retiring! When people comment on your look, you have brought interest and beauty to your immediate surroundings. Good for you!

Accessories are your friends. Nothing defines your look so much as your "finish." As a second-fifty-year woman, do not fret too much about proper scale. If you are a small woman, a bold accessory will get you compliments. This is not your shrinking-violet stage of life. This is your dahlia stage of life! Stand tall and stand out. It feels good.

Preaccessorized Clothing

What if you don't wear jewelry but understand the value of accessorizing to bring attention back to your face? You can effectively use embroidered blouses or T-shirts. Many tops have beautiful details leading the eye to the face and surrounding the neck. T-shirts may have artistic cutout treatments that look like a separate necklace. These items are "preaccessorized." They really do not need another separate piece of jewelry to define them or you. They meet your goal of presenting "eye candy," something to savor, around the face.

Yes, accessories are dessert. If you wear *only* accessories you will end up in jail. (But what a great finish!) They are sweets that you get to have and enjoy over and over. They seldom "don't fit," and they keep for years. Collect, save, and revisit your accessories often.

There is a greater chance that you wear too few accessories than you wear too many. The following checklist is a fun way for you and your friends to dissect and improve your current looks. This exercise is for fun, not judgment. A second-fifty-year woman is able to understand that differences are to be embraced, not booed.

Fashion Balance Scorecard

Are you a Natural/Sporty or a proverbial Drama Queen? The beauty of it is that you can play all the roles in the privacy of your own home. Maybe you are a closet Dramatic and didn't know it!

Fashion Balance Scorecard
Rate Your Pizzazz
Too little? Too much? Or just right?

Score 1 point for each
   (or 2 points for something especially outstanding)

____	Each visible piece of clothing
____	Each accent color
____	Each patterned fabric
____	Each high-textured fabric
____	Each accent trim
____	Decorative buttons
____	Each piece of jewelry
____	"Set" hairdo
____	Eyeglasses
____	Colored or "French" nails
____	Patterned socks
____	Colored hose
____	Funky shoes
____	TOTAL

Did you score between 8 and 15?
   If so, then walk with confidence! You put just the right amount of thought into your dressing today!

Did you score below 8?
   If so, you may be dangerously close to boring. Add some pizzazz!

Did you score over 14?
   If so, you're what's commonly referred to as a Drama Queen! Keep them guessing!

Glasses as Accessories

Glasses are often the companion of a second-fifty-year woman. They are a very important part of your signature look. Prescription glasses are expensive. If you own only one pair, echo your hair color to best complement your face.

A bold frame is a personal choice. Some women use sunglass frames for their regular lenses very effectively. These frames are heavier and the physical presence of these women, when they walk into a room, is commanding. Think Sally Jesse Raphael and her oversized red-framed set or Edith Head and her bold, black frames. See how easily you remember their look? It can be yours!

Some women have multiple pairs of glasses in colors from red to purple to tortoiseshell. They dress to complement the color of these glasses and their look literally brings all the attention back to their eyes. If it is in your budget and you have a favorite color you wear often, investing in a second pair of glasses to coordinate with that color could be one of your best accessory choices.

Accessorizing Your Feet

Second-fifty-year women eventually give up three-inch heels for more comfortable footwear. In no way does this mean that the foot cannot draw attention.

Adding a dramatic shoe design or color to a neutral outfit may be all that is needed to bring up the conversation level. Women love interesting shoes. Spotlighting shoes is especially fun if there is a great story behind your having found them. Were you on vacation or were they hidden on the wrong size rack?

A second way to accessorize feet inexpensively is with funky socks. Some women collect them by the hundreds. Don't be afraid to venture into the sock aisle looking for something that echoes your totem or announces something that you collect or maybe some unusual color you wear. Socks are an easy way to reveal a little something about your personality and why someone should want to get to know you. They are especially great for different holidays. You know you have hit your sweet spot with your sock choice when your grandchildren are enthralled with them. Let novelty footwear give you happy feet!

Smile

From head to toe, your accessories should still feature you being just you. The final and best accessory to any outfit is your smile. Remember, your smile is one of your two most defining features. Make sure that it shines. There is nothing quite as youthful as a bright smile. To brighten yours, you may choose to try the new over-the-counter teeth whiteners available at your grocery or pharmacy or invest in the new light systems at your dentist's office.

A woman with a sunny outlook and ready smile is more attractive than one who doesn't smile as much at any age but especially during the second fifty years. Keep it simple. Smile!

Sometimes the aging process leaves one with a stern or dour expression. If your facial features droop, turning your relaxed lip line downward, make a concerted effort to add a small, smirklike upturn to your look. Check yourself out in the mirror. Practice so you know how this half-smile feels when you are out and about. It worked for Whistler's mother. Let it work for you.

Smiles are free. Send them at will. What a perfect signature look!

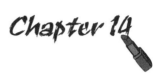

Chapter 14

Color Me Here:
Reversing the Aging Dilemma

As noted in chapter 2, just when you have gotten so much experience and have so many answers about the issues of living, nature plays a cruel joke. Your hair starts to lose its color and your skin tone becomes less vibrant. Eventually your step slows and the world goes rushing by, unaware of the vast accumulation of knowledge you hold. You have lost the "presence" of youth.

This is one of those "just get over it" facts of life. Do not dwell on your eventuality but plan through it. The counterbalance to losing natural vibrancy is simply *color*. Color is power for the second-fifty-year woman. Nature uses color to gain attention and denote beauty. Nature is not afraid to be lavish and bold. Nature loves hues and has little regard for the perfect match. So should you!

From Peahen to Peacock

It is time to cease being a peahen and become a peacock. What-ever your color choices in your first fifty years, you must double your boldness now. If you are the friend of a Dramatic who jumps at the chance to increase her already formidable presence, you may need to steer her directly to the next section. But if you fall into the majority—the quietly put-together woman—it is time to purposefully plan to embolden your look.

If you have been "color draped," you have some idea of your best colors—for the period in which you were draped. Your color needs change as you change. If you are more com-fortable with a prescribed formula, be redraped every five years. Skin tones can change that much. I personally cannot be held to specific reds, blues, and purples; I find the color sys-tems informative but confining. I also do not agree that one must soften one's color palette as one ages. We need more color now, not less.

The following discussion is based on my experience with beautifully dressed older women who get frequent compli-ments on their look. Some of their choices may fly in the face of the "rules," but they are great role models for your choices.

Color Basics

First, some colors are hard for nearly any second-fifty-year woman to wear with full confidence. These difficult colors are those positioned on the color wheel closest to your skin tone, the yellow and orange ranges. Wear these only after profes-sional assessment. Your "can do no wrong" colors are directly across the wheel from yellow and orange: blue, purple, and blue-green.

Second, if you don't fight Mother Nature, follow her lead. If your gray hair is silver white, white is your basic color. If your hair is ivory, then soft white or winter white is your basic color (year-round). If you have perfect salt-and-pepper colored hair, you can wear gray, black, and white very effectively. The goal is to frame your face.

Your hair is the natural frame for the top and sides of your face. Echo that color in your blouse or top and you will come into focus.

Whether it's natural or "done," your hair color is your own. If you color your hair, dress to that hair color. You may be a blonde for the first time in your life. Good for you! According to Joanna Pitman, author of *On Blondes*, you have made a great choice. For starters, she says, "people see blondes as having lots of youthful vitality, and being blonde may make you look younger. Since babies and children tend to have lighter hair than adults do, there is a subtle correlation between youth and blondness. Golden-locked girls are also seen as the most wealthy and glamorous, both because gold equals money in our collective unconscious and because getting your hair lightened by a professional generally costs a lot."[1]

So now that you are blonde, make your basic color soft white, not pure white, no matter what you used to wear. When you wear prints, look for a background that is ivory, not white. I have found that since bleaching streaks in my hair, my "winter" palette no longer rules my look. I can now wear rich earth tones effectively for the first time.

If your hair color varies on a monthly basis, you may need several "basic" wardrobes. The rule, such as it is, is to honor your hair color and you will be seen.

If you dye your hair red, you are using the rarest of colors. True redheads constitute no more than 2 percent of the world population.[2] Red hair draws attention. Good for you! As a redhead, look for clothing that echoes your exact color somewhere in the print. You will look particularly fabulous if you can find a rich auburn top in your exact hair color.

As discussed in the last chapter, whatever your hair color, purchase an accessory wardrobe that repeats it. When in doubt about your clothing or your accessories, default to your hair color. It is never wrong. Wear these basics and you will shine.

Whether your hair is white, salt-and-pepper, blonde, red, or warm brunette, wearing your hair color from head to toe, including accessories, presents one of your most powerful looks. Starting there, you can freely add other colors or prints over your basics. With your best colors next to your face, you are free to wear what you love. You should, in the end, have your default color represented in multiple pieces in your closet.

The Eyes Have It

Your second "natural" best color repeats your eye color. If you have rich brown eyes and hair, nature assures that wearing a rich brown will showcase your assets. If your eyes are blue, violet, green, or hazel, you will know you have hit your stride when what you wear makes your eyes shine in a way that people notice.

Sometimes customers comment, "Here I go, buying something blue again. Maybe I should put this back and buy another color."

If this is your dilemma, the answer is absolutely not. If your comfort zone is blue, stick with blue. This is your signature color. If you have blue eyes and prefer blue wardrobe pieces, you have subconsciously gravitated to your best color.

Having a closet full of multiple tones and intensities of your best and favorite colors gives you plenty of range to express yourself. If blue is your signature, have powder blue, electric blue, and navy plus many blues in between. Adding another color to your wardrobe just for the sake of adding another color does not justify the purchase. You most likely will not wear this item or will feel out of place when you do. Use a color only when it makes you look *and* feel fabulous.

I equate this to going to Baskin Robbins for my favorite ice cream, Jamoca Almond Fudge. The times I have not been true to my taste for ice cream and have felt I should try another flavor have always ended in disappointment. I indeed spoiled the occasion. I derive pleasure from my taste, both for ice cream and clothing. I am happiest and therefore most confident when I honor my taste. Honoring your taste is in your best interest too. When it comes to clothes (or ice cream), always buy your favorite "flavor."

Wearing multiple intensities of your best color makes an effective statement also. A bold tone in a jacket with a pastel tone for the blouse presents an interesting take on monochromatic dressing. When possible, purchase pants and basic top combinations together to facilitate a mix-and-match closet.

You do not need to have a perfect understanding of color to feel confident in your look. Use these few tricks and look like a pro. Now dressing is easy and you are not only good-looking but looking good! You will be seen.

Part III
<u>Playing It Forward:</u> Your Legacy

*Y*ou validated and loved yourself and learned to *Be*.
You had fun dressing the part and being *Seen*.

It is time to make a difference. It is time to complete the circle.

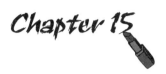

Chapter 15

Compliments: Completing the Circle

*T*his book opened with the stated goal for you to be seen. You have perhaps found a few hints within these pages that let your inner girl play dress-up as well as be a bit of a show-off. Remember, this is not your second childhood but actually your first because you now engage in play on purpose. If you have found that several of the secrets from the sisterhood have opened your eyes and increased your excitement about your second fifty years, then this book has succeeded. You have applied these principles to your own self-image and played at creating your public persona. You have also had a few moments *being seen* that have been life affirming.

I promised earlier that I would address completing the circle of experience from loving oneself unconditionally to holding all others in warm regard. There is one very simple way to enrich the world around you and receive the same riches in return. This process is completely self-sustained and guaranteed to fill your life to the brim. You will need to interact with other individuals, but you get to instigate interactions at will. The reward is plain magic.

And just what is this magic elixir, this richest secret of the sisterhood? Compliments—both received and given—are the mother lode of riches in our second fifty years.

Recall the endorphin response addressed in relation to shopping? Endorphins leave you with a sense of well-being, relieve pain, increase the immune system's ability to protect you, and make you feel just like being in love. Well, there is even more good news! That same endorphin surge is the hidden gift wrapped in a sincere compliment, both one that is given and one that is received. This gift is available anytime you have contact with another human being. Even more profoundly, it is available every time you revisit the experience in your mind. This surge of endorphins can be your God-given drug of choice. You have full permission to be high on life!

Compliment University: Receiving 101

If you are uncomfortable when someone says something wonderful about you, you are not alone. You have had years to compare yourself to "perfect" role models and are very aware that you are probably at best just average. Now you are older and that youthful beauty is looking further and further removed from your vision. If you still feel these sentences apply to you, get posthaste back to the front of the book. (If you don't understand yet how beautiful you truly are, you need to revisit part 1.)

Because of what you've learned here, you are now empowered. There are no wallflowers in the sisterhood. You will be seen. Being seen means that compliments will come your way and you must be ready to properly receive them.

Receiving compliments properly is an art, the mark of a lady. This takes practice, practice, practice. For instance, if someone says to you, "Wow! You look fabulous," how do you respond? Without flinching, without even thinking, your immediate response should be a resounding, "Why *thank* you!" Or possibly, "Thank yooouuu!" Physically, put your whole body into the acceptance of these kind words. Lean slightly toward the speaker and smile wide-eyed. Emotionally hug the compliment. Keep your response very, very appreciative and warm. Reward the sender of compliments with your instant and joyful acceptance.

If you are truly uncomfortable with accepting a particular compliment, an acceptable alternative is, "Thank you for saying so." This allows you permission to work through your internal doubts without rejecting someone's gracious words. Never diminish the gift by responding, "Oh, this old thing," or with other compliment-diverting mumbles.

Emotionally hugging a compliment means you are ready to accept all the endorphin rewards your system has to offer. With practice, the effect gets stronger and stronger. Hugging the compliment means that you do not question it, deny it, or add your own dose of reality to it. You learn to accept compliments at face value. Remember the old adage, "Don't look a gift horse in the mouth." Denying a compliment spoils the fun, and compliments should be a fun part of our existence. You will know you understand the concept when you give your compliments a bear hug because they feel so good. Let a compliment wash over your soul. Appreciate being seen.

Something very special happens when an honest compliment is sincerely embraced. When you enthusiastically acknowledge compliments, you give a wonderful gift back to the senders—their own dose of endorphins! What a wonderful gift of nature that our wiring is meant to connect full circle. The giver of the endorphin surge becomes the receiver. The process costs nothing and it gives double.

Promise to *never* deflect a compliment again. If you protest, you deny the senders their reward and make them feel foolish. How unkind. You owe your compliment givers an enthusiastic thank-you.

Compliment University: Giving 101

You must be good at accepting compliments to be good at giving them. You need to know what hugging compliments feels like so you can see others feel hugged by your words. What if no one compliments you? Are you stuck waiting until someone does? Therein lies the beauty of compliments. You can start the circle yourself by making kind comments to those around you. It may be to store clerks , church members, or strangers on the street. This should not be a forced process or it will seem phony. Your compliments must be honest. How can you be sure? There is one simple test of an honest compliment.

Honest Compliments

Nothing rings more hollow than a pandering comment. How can you be sure that your compliments are honest? Giving an honest compliment is this easy: *if you think it in passing, say it.* Speak your musings. That's all. How many times do you pass someone on the sidewalk and notice something nice about her look but never say a word? Positive judgments of a beautiful world need to be spoken. A wonderful thought floats through your mind and you simply open your mouth and say what you think out loud. To perfect strangers? Especially to perfect strangers!

A compliment is a life-affirming statement. It shows that we see something outstanding about someone else. We recognize the effort they have taken to *be seen*. A compliment shows that we believe in being seen. No other gift is as giving and potentially life changing.

My own story speaks to the power of the unexpected compliment. You see, *I am a stunning creature*. This assessment is not open to your vote or to public opinion. It is a fact I will take to my grave. Let me tell you how I know.

It was a rare sunny spring day in Portland, Oregon. The year was 1992 and I was forty-four years old. I was walking up a path to deliver a package to one of my customers and moved to one side to allow an older woman to pass. As she reached me, she said, "My, you are a stunning creature." I was so taken aback I literally stopped. Then, hugging her compliment, I responded emphatically, "Oh, my! Thank you so much!" We both proceeded on our way, never to meet again.

In retrospect, that "older woman" was probably about the age I am today. I am sure she has absolutely no idea the value of the gift she gave me that day. More than ten years later, I vividly remember her comment. I am still hugging her compliment. Because of that stranger's kind words, I will live the rest of my life as a "stunning creature."

What she could not know was my personal history and the huge impact her simply verbalizing her thought would have on my life. You see, I am the daughter of a truly stunning mother. Mom grew up in the Teton Mountains of Wyoming and in her teens was a calendar model who posed with championship quarter horses. She was courted by New York modeling agencies and Hollywood, but those careers did not appeal to her.

My dad, whom I love to distraction, met and married my mom in college. He is a wonderful man. What he is not is stunning. As a young child, I actually thought he rather resembled Jiminy Cricket.

At about four years of age, I distinctly remember walking with my dad, reaching up to hold his hand as we walked through a crowd. Old friends of my dad's on more than one occasion would say, "My, she's your spittin' image!" Now, even at that young age, I knew that that meant "poor child." It meant I had the genetic potential to be an unusual beauty like my mother but was not.

On the day that unknown woman gave a stranger the gift of her compliment, she undid all those years of comparison. I stood alone as a stunning creature! I am still a stunning creature. I will be a stunning creature until I die. If you don't think you have ever seen a stunning seventy-, eighty-, or ninety-year-old, just watch me. I will be stunning because I became stunning in 1992. It is now my state of being, a gift that cannot be taken from me. Thank you, dear lady on the sidewalk, wherever you are.

How often do we not verbalize compliments because we assume that the person we have noticed probably hears what we have to say all the time? Don't be the judge of that. Say the kind things you think. You just may be giving someone a gift that they sorely need. Don't budget your compliments. Remember: *if you think it, say it*!

What if you are shy? What if you have always watched life from the sidelines? How do you now move to center stage and be seen and heard as you give compliments?

Compliment University: Assignments

First, I want to compliment you: if you have read this far, you are a superior student. You have shown that you want to be taught positive ways to relate within your sphere. But how do you learn to become comfortable with both giving and receiving honest compliments? This section, which is self-paced but supportive, will show you how.

Compliment Your Friends

One of the first and best places to practice giving and receiving compliments is with your current circle of friends. Get together for lunch and spend an hour saying kind things about each other. What first attracted you to each other? What positive elements do you each bring to the relationships? How has knowing each other enriched your individual lives? You will find this a very intimate exercise and one that leaves each of you enriched beyond your wildest expectations. If you think it, say it! Start with those you already love.

Another good place to start spreading goodwill is among those who serve you on a regular basis at grocery stores, department stores, or restaurants. Clerks and servers are often under stress and a kind acknowledgment of something personal that attracted you to their line or table goes a long way to making their day special. It does not take long before you see that they anticipate your trip through their line. Their eyes light up and they sincerely love to see you!

Compliment Strangers

Complimenting strangers may sound odd. Again, if you think something nice, just say it. Then keep walking. Think of it as "hit and run" complimenting! Have a kind thought, pause to express it, then move on before the receiver of your compliment can comment.

Any kind thought will do. "My, you have beautiful hair" (or hands, eyes, legs, teeth—whatever you noted). Notice what quality about someone takes on a life of its own and becomes a fully formed thought without your consciously trying. You can mention accessories, clothing, cars, children, anything that made you stop and notice. Sometimes the greatest compliment is "My, what a beautiful family." Just acknowledge that you have seen someone else. Remember, see and be seen!

The easiest way to practice complimenting strangers is to begin by doing it silently. Become aware when you are thinking something nice about another human being. Find a bench at a mall or some other high-traffic area and people-watch. What do you first notice about the people you see? What is striking about each one? Are you aware of judgmental thoughts? Turn them around. Remember, it is our differences that make us special. Work at this until you find that positive thoughts are coming almost automatically. Now check your own mood. Feeling high, aren't you? You see, even silent compliments give you a positive chemical reaction. Soon enough, you feel bursting with personal joy and will just naturally let slip those kind thoughts you are holding. You will become verbal when you become so full of compliments you absolutely *have* to share them. Trust me! What you speak will be the truth and will make someone else's day a little more special.

Compliment Older Women

Now step beyond your normal interaction patterns and do something on purpose. Specifically notice one of your older "sisters." You have already addressed the issue of disappearing as you get older, and you agree you don't want your sisters ignored. Many older women not only fight disappearing, but as widows they are missing the closeness of human touch and caring that they shared with their husbands. Imagine the aloneness they feel. When you notice one of your older sisters and lightly engage her inner girl, you not only see her, you touch her. It is so easy to acknowledge her emotional hunger. I guarantee that she will bear-hug the attention. The compliment does not have to be long or involved. Just let her know she has not disappeared in your eyes. Notice her smile, her hair, her nails, or maybe a rich color she is wearing. Compliment what is obviously a strength. You see, someday, if you are very lucky, it will be your turn to be the older sister. Do unto others.

Compliment Younger Women

Now take all this practice in compliment giving to a level you may not think is necessary. Compliment *young* women. Your immediate feeling may be that they would not value your thoughts. Be assured, they need all the positive reinforcement they can get. In my youth, the archetypical teen was Annette Funicello—beautiful, soft, sweet, feminine, and virginal. She set an almost unattainable goal. Today, young women are expected to define their identity against that of Britney Spears or Pamela Anderson. Older women complete the circle when they bring their view of positive living and self-loving to those who, like we did before them, need a little boost in self-esteem.

Support the Young

With the advantage of your years, can you not look at today's twentysomethings and ask, "Are they not all beautiful?" From the perspective of the second fifty years, youth *is* beauty. Did you feel confidently beautiful in your twenties? *No.* Guess what? Neither do today's young women. The world is so competitive. The young have no better sense of self than we did at their age. They benefit significantly from unexpected compliments given by us older women passing through their sphere. We need to share the wealth and the knowledge of our understanding. We need to see and be seen.

I had a wonderful young intake nurse for one of my recreational surgery stints. We laughed and had a wonderful time with the process of getting ready. In one preoperative phone call, I said in passing, "What would you know? You are so beautiful!" I made this statement not as a compliment but as an obvious fact.

There was a moment of silence on the line and then she made one of the saddest comments I have ever heard: "That is the first time anyone has ever told me I was beautiful."

I did a quick inventory in my mind. She was a big woman, tall and solid with beautiful dark eyes and hair. Was this nurse the quintessential California beach-blonde bombshell? No, but she was a beauty nonetheless. I told her that I used the word "beautiful" as an appropriate adjective and to accept it as so because I only give honest compliments. What was wrong with her parents, I wondered, to never tell her she was beautiful? Was hers a classic case of having a prettier sister?

My words to her meant she had permission to see herself as a beauty in her own right. I hope she carries that belief within herself as her personal truth from now on.

After that, guess who made sure to come say hi every time she saw my name on the schedule? And why not? She stood alone as a beauty with me. All previous comparisons others had made dropped away. We became members of each other's fan club.

See and be seen. Surround yourself with your fans. Challenge yourself daily to ask

Have I complimented someone older?
Have I complimented someone younger?
Have I complimented a stranger?
Have I complimented a friend?
Have I complimented my family?

Imagine a world where everyone gave three compliments every day. What a wonderful world. Remember, the giver becomes the receiver. In this game, you cannot lose!

You may be familiar with the phrase "pay it forward." As a member of the sisterhood there is an inner girl twist: You *play* it forward by complimenting your older sisters. You play it behind by complimenting younger women. And you play it beside you to your companions and acquaintances. Complimenting is as easy as having a positive thought and sharing it immediately. The rewards are enormous. With your compliments, you gently change the flow of an individual life—maybe for a moment, maybe for a lifetime. You cannot begin to know the depth of self-doubt you remove and the power you instill. See and be seen. I know this is true because I am a stunning creature.

Just say it.

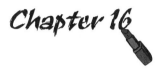

Chapter 16

I Want to Get Old:
The Power of the Mind

*E*mbedded thoughts become true. Whatsoever a woman thinks, so is she. The power of positive or negative thinking has been proven over and over.

You have started to plan for your second fifty years. How do you plan for possibly frail years? Will you really want to get older when you are truly old? How can you know?

When you honor the process and keep moving to the best of your ability, life is good. How do I know? I offer you two stories.

Boots

A wonderful, inspiring woman embodies all that can be true for the latter part of your second fifty years. She resides in an independent retirement community that is served by a traveling boutique. When the boutique is set up for a day of shopping at her community, this lovely lady must traverse the length of a large apartment complex to shop. She starts early so she can pick her favorite new outfit and still return to her apartment for lunch.

This would not be a particularly noteworthy event except for one fact. Her steps are very slow and her stride is short. In fact, she would probably refer to her gait as a shuffle. She sports a walker to assure her balance. In other words, her trip to the boutique is accomplished with great effort.

This picture should change your perception of her journey. It should not change your perception of her attitude toward life. You see, for the whole time it takes her to reach the boutique to buy herself something wonderful, she keeps repeating to herself over and over, "Keep moving, boots, just keep moving, boots." This is her mantra. You can guess her nickname—Boots.

Boots honors her abilities. Boots is not ashamed to have grown old. Boots does not quit or just sit in her apartment. She is having a good time. Boots does not want your sympathy, but she will gladly accept your high regard.

From her I have learned that I can expect to "keep moving" with whatever parts are still moving. Everything between then and now is all good. That is the inspiration of Boots!

But what if you become completely bedridden? Should you despair? Ask Mary.

Mary Christian

In actuality, you can't talk to Mary because she died recently—as the longest-living American at 113. Her obituary speaks to us about living so long.[1]

First, she lived at home until around the age of 103! For the last year of her life, she was bedridden, nearly blind, and hard of hearing. If you think she wished she could die, you are wrong, so wrong. She loved the recognition her "oldest American" status brought and loved to talk to reporters about her early childhood memories. She loved being *seen*.

She had a reputation as a strong-willed, independent woman to the end. According to her niece, Mary had made up her mind she was going to be 114. Although she did not make it, her spirit lives on in our understanding that her inner girl accompanied her to her grave. Mary kept planning for one more year—even at 113.

The Danger of Being Alone

It has been proven that effective care without affective touching is terminal to the human spirit. Babies in orphanages may be well cared for, but if they are left alone, denied human contact, not only do they not thrive, they die.

The need for human touch does not diminish with age. How important it is to reach out to those older than yourself. Great age means a person has had familial losses, whether of children or a spouse. Humans were created to touch one another. Reach out to those ahead of you on the aging spectrum. As many of us band together, providing love and attention to those ahead of us, the world will be changed.

One reward is immediate because you have connected with another human being. But you will have an even greater, more egocentric, reward. If you help change the world, there will be strong women reaching forward to you when it is your time.

Epilogue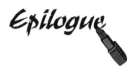

Best Wishes

The book opened with planning to see and be seen. I hope the world and your place in it have gained a richness of purpose and human interaction that will make your second fifty years (or whatever portion you have left) your most powerful.

Wish for a long, straightforward path into old age. Do not deny that there will be various health issues and personal losses to deal with. These are detours from the path, not the path itself. Health issues do not define your life and your value. Find support from others along any detour you are called to take. Then get back on this wonderful path to living, not dying, into old age. That is the power of strategic aging. That is the power of aging with a vengeance. That is the power of the sisterhood.

Affirm these words to yourself: I will live long. I will live well. I will be seen. I will make a difference. And, finally, I will be missed.

With gratitude I acknowledge the many second-fifty-year women who have shared with me the joy of a long life and the joy of costuming. From them I learned the simplest strategy to a well-lived life and the fulfillment of our highest purpose.

Be seen! Make a difference!

Appendix

Resources

Organizations

AICI (Association of Image Consultants International)
International Headquarters
12300 Ford Road, Suite 135
Dallas, TX 75234
972-755-1503
www.aici.org

> AICI is a "non-profit professional association of men and women specializing in visual appearance." It is a great source for finding a personal shopper or image coach.

Sweet Potato Queens
Jackson, Mississippi
601-366-0770
www.sweetpotatoqueens.com

> Fun-loving groups of women organized by author Jill Browne.

The Red Hat Society
431 S. Acacia Avenue
Fullerton, CA 92831
714-738-0001
www.redhatsociety.com

> *"The place where there is fun after fifty (and before) for women of all walks of life."*

Women's Shelters

Contact your local crisis intervention service or women's resource center. The locations of the shelters must be kept secret for security reasons, but drop-offs can be arranged.

Also, check your yellow pages for local senior services and organizations.

Recommended Reading List

Beauty

Nix-Rice, Nancy. *Looking Good*. Portland, OR: Palmer/Pletsch Publishing, 1996.

> *A comprehensive guide to wardrobe planning, color, and personal style development.*

Pooser, Doris. *Always In Style*. Menlo Park, CA: Crisp Publications, 1997.

> *The acclaimed classic on creating your personal style, including hair and makeup.*

Spillane, Mary. *Branding Yourself.* London: Pan Books, 2000.

This book was written for businesswomen but translates well to life in general.

Health

Morris, Barbara, R.Ph. *Boomers Really Can Put Old on Hold.* Escondido, CA: Image F/X Publishing, 2002.

This second-fifty-year pharmacist understands and lives what she preaches.

Northrup, Christine, M.D. *The Wisdom of Menopause: Creating Physical and Emotional Health and Healing during the Change.* New York: Bantam Dell Publishing, 2001.

Northrup, Christine, M.D. *Women's Bodies, Women's Wisdom: Creating Physical and Emotional Health and Healing.* New York: Bantam Dell Publishing, 2002.

Dr. Northrup should be read by every woman planning for a long, healthy life.

The Physicians Desk Reference Family Guide Encyclopedia of Medical Care. New York: Ballantine Books, 1999.

The book doctors use to find out what ails you.

Waterhouse, Debra. *Outsmarting the Midlife Fat Cell: Winning Weight Control Strategies for Woman over 35 to Stay Fit through Menopause.* New York: Hyperion Press, 1999.

Diet centers do not speak to the reality of the second-fifty-year body. This book does.

National Institutes of Health. "Calculate Your Body Mass Index," www.nhlbisupport.com/bmi.

Using the BMI calculator, adjust your weight figure to see how much weight you need to lose to reduce your BMI.

Personal Growth

Bradley, John, Russ Korth, and Jay Carty. *Discovering Your Natural Talents: How to Love What You Do and Do What You Love.* Colorado Springs: NavPress, 1994.

Find your highest and best use. Your heart will sing.

Bradshaw, John. *Homecoming: Reclaiming and Championing Your Inner Child.* New York: Doubleday, 1992.

Reparent yourself into an emotionally healthy second fifty years.

Dwight, Eleanor. *Diana Vreeland.* New York: William Morrow, 2002.

An inspirational story of how to go from ordinary to extraordinary.

Hendrix, Harville. *Getting the Love You Want.* New York: Henry Holt & Company, 1988.

Be loved. How to know when it is healthy.

Kaputa, Catherine. "The Power of Self Brand," http://www.selfbrand.com.

Making an Impact

Laroche, Loretta. *Life Is Short—Wear Your Party Pants: Ten Simple Truths That Lead to an Amazing Life.* Carlsbad, CA: Hay House, 2003.

Wearing party pants alone will make your day!

Lerner, Harriet. *The Dance of Anger: A Woman's Guide to Changing the Patterns of Intimate Relationships.* New York: Quill, 1997.

Lerner, Harriet. *The Dance of Intimacy: A Woman's Guide to Courageous Acts of Change in Key Relationships.* New York: Perennial, 1997.

Learn where you fit in the puzzle of relationships.

McGraw, Phillip C. *Self Matters: Creating Your Life from the Inside Out.* New York: Simon and Schuster, 2001.

Do it because you can. Straight talk on defining yourself.

Notes

CHAPTER 1: LIFE JOURNEY: BEING BORN IS TERMINAL

1. "Positively Life-Extending," *More*, February 2003, 122.
2. Frank Darabout, *The Shawshank Redemption*, Castle Rock Studios, 1994.
3. Sharon Begley, "Getting Inside a Teen Brain, "*Newsweek*, February 28, 2000, 58. Sharon Begley, "Mind Expansion: Inside the Teen-age Brain," *Newsweek*, May 8, 2000, 68.
4. Debra Waterhouse, *Outsmarting the Midlife Fat Cell: Winning Weight Control Strategies for Women over 35 to Stay Fit through Menopause* (New York: Hyperion, 1999).
5. Dr. Annette Colby, "Body Testing: Is the Body Mass Index Really Accurate?" *Health and Wellness*, February 2003, 34–35.
6. Don Freeman, "Hirschfield Lived Life the Way He Drew It: With Elegance and Style," *San Diego Union-Tribune*, January 22, 2003.
7. Obituary, *San Diego Union-Tribune*, July 6, 2003.

CHAPTER 2: AGEISM: GETTING BEYOND "OLD"

1. John Bradshaw, *Homecoming: Reclaiming and Championing Your Inner Child* (New York: Doubleday, 1992).
2. U.S. Census Bureau, "Table 1. Population by Age, Sex, Race and Historic Origin: March 2002," http://www.census.gov/polulation/socdemo/age/ppl-167/tab01.xls.

CHAPTER 3: STARTING ON THE INSIDE: DEVELOPING
A PASSION FOR YOUR FUTURE

1. Bette Midler, interview by Barbara Walters, 1980, "Bette Midler Video Archives," http://bettemidleraloha.com/bette.htm.

CHAPTER 4: STRATEGIC PLANNING: IT'S NOT JUST FOR BUSINESS

1. Catherine Kaputa, "The Power of Self Brand," *The Art of Branding*, http://www.selfbrand.com.
2. Ibid.

CHAPTER 5: SELF LOVE: MAKING IT UNCONDITIONAL

1. Eleanor Dwight, "Becoming Diana Vreeland," *Victoria*, November 2002, 38–41.
2. Ibid.
3 Ibid.
4. John Bradley, Russ Korth, and Jay Carty, *Discovering Your Natural Talents: How to Love What You Do and Do What You Love* (Colorado Springs: NavPress, 1994).

CHAPTER 6: OTHER LOVE: OFFERING WARM REGARD

1. Harville Hendrix, *Getting the Love You Want* (New York: Henry Holt, 1988).
2. "Depression," http://www.healthsquare.com. Accessed 8/28/03, article no longer available.

CHAPTER 7: THE SCIENCE OF SHOPPING

1. "Why We Shop" and "How They Sell," *Buyology*, The Learning Channel, November 30, 2001.
2. Marilyn Albert and Guy McKhann, "Keep Your Brain Young," *Wall Street Journal*, July 8, 2002.
3. Ibid.

CHAPTER 8: PLAYING DRESS-UP: WHAT YOU SEE IS WHAT YOU GET

1. Jennifer Alfano, "Ralph's Rules of Attraction," *Harper's Bazaar*, December 2002, 146.

CHAPTER 10: THE PERSONALITY OF DRESSING: COSTUMING FOR YOUR BRAND

1. Mary Spillane, *Branding Yourself* (London: Pan Books, 2000), 163.

CHAPTER 11: FLATTERING STYLE: TRICKS FOR THE SECOND FIFTY YEARS

1. *Belle of the Nineties*, Universal Studios, 1934.

CHAPTER 13: EYE CANDY: ACCESSORIZING TO AMAZE

1.   *Webster's New World Dictionary*, 2nd ed. (New York, Pocketbooks, 2002).

CHAPTER 14: COLOR ME HERE: REVERSING THE AGING DILEMMA

1.   "What Your Hair Color Says about You," *Cosmopolitan*, March 2003, 195–198.
2.   Ibid.

CHAPTER 16: I WANT TO GET OLD: THE POWER OF THE MIND

1.   Obituary, *San Diego Union-Tribune*, April 27, 2003.

Index

About the Author

*W*hen Claudia Jean enters a room, she fills it with a striking sense of style and confidence, not to mention a passionate view on aging with a vengeance. A nationally recognized authority on fashion, a powerful marketing executive, a successful entrepreneur, and an endearing public speaker, Claudia Jean has been addressing the issue of fashion for the "over-junior" market for more than a decade.

Claudia Jean's no-nonsense approach to the female form and the issues of dressing it help audiences feel confident about their bodies and the clothes they wear.

Since the debut of her company, The CLAUDIA JEAN Collection (www.claudiajean.com), in 1997, she has helped thousands of women transform their sense of style, filling closets with clothes that flatter the figure and enhance self-esteem. Her powerful, insightful approach cuts through the preconceived notions of a youth-obsessed society. Inspired by the thousands of women she has helped develop a unique fashion style, Claudia Jean has realized a personal passion for living long and well.